The FLEXIBLE FODMAP DIET COOKBOOK

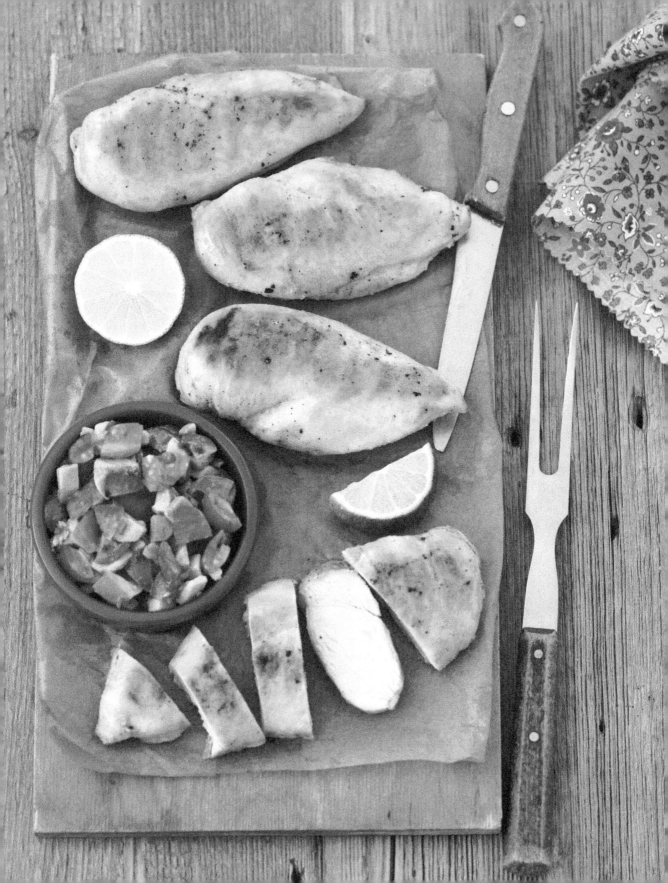

The Flexible FODMAP DIET COOKBOOK

Customizable Low-FODMAP Meal Plans & Recipes for a Symptom-Free Life

Laura Manning, RD & Karen Frazier

ROCKRIDGE
PRESS

This book is dedicated to my family: For John, my husband, for always
encouraging me and for putting up with my hectic schedule. And to both of
my children, Lily and Johnny, for always trying and eating everything I cook.

—Laura

For Jim and Tanner, who have put up with my unique dietary needs
for nearly two decades.

—Karen

For general information on our other products and services or to obtain technical support, please contact our Customer Care Department within the United States (866) 744-2665, or outside the United States at (510) 253-0500.

Rockridge Press publishes its books in a variety of electronic and print formats. Some content that appears in print may not be available in electronic books, and vice versa.

Cover photography © Stockfood/Leigh Beisch, Stocksy/ Ruth Black, Stocksy/Harold Walker, Stockfood/Magdalena Hendey

Interior photography © Stockfood/RuaCastilho, p.2; Stockfood/Ina Peters, p.6; Stockfood/Gräfe & Unzer Verlag/mona binner PHOTOGRAPHIE, p.12; Stockfood/ Rua Castilho, p.32; Stockfood/PhotoCuisine/Phillippe Asset, p.58; Stockfood/Magdalena Hendey, p.76; Stockfood/Magdalena Hendey, p.94; Stockfood/Jalag/ Maike Jessen, p.112; Stockfood/Leigh Beisch, p.134; Stockfood/John Hay, p.158; Stockfood/Gareth Morgans, p.176; Stockfood/Rua Castilho, p.188

ISBN: Print 978-1-62315-818-7 | eBook 978-1-62315-819-4

BEFORE TRYING
A LOW-FODMAP DIET

If you're ready to start a low-FODMAP diet to help control your irritable bowel syndrome (IBS) symptoms, consider the following:

The low-FODMAP diet is a *temporary* diet designed to calm your digestive system. In general, people need to follow this diet for 2 to 6 weeks to calm symptoms. FODMAP is a hefty acronym that stands for fermentable oligosaccharides, disaccharides, monosaccharides, and polyols, or certain carbohydrates in food that some people cannot digest easily.

During the calming phase, it is important that you eliminate all FODMAPs. Your digestive system needs special care so it can heal itself. To do this, you will avoid all FODMAPs for several weeks. Consuming FODMAPs during this calming phase can cause irritation and flare-ups. It is important that during the early phases of the plan, you maintain strict control over your diet.

You can customize the diet. Once your digestive system calms down, you'll begin the process of reintroducing foods and food groups into your diet to determine which foods you can eat and still remain symptom-free and which foods you need to avoid.

There are four types of meal plans included.

B A **BASIC** low-FODMAP meal plan for IBS

A A low-fat, low-acid, low-FODMAP meal plan for IBS plus **ACID REFLUX** or GERD (gastroesophageal reflux disease)

C A high-fiber, low-FODMAP meal plan for **IBS-C** (constipation-predominant)

D A low-fiber, low-FODMAP plan with modified food textures for **IBS-D** (diarrhea-predominant) or **IBD** in remission

You can choose the plan that most closely fits your symptoms.

Talk with your primary health-care provider. Anytime you start a new way of eating, it is important to talk with your health-care provider and a registered dietitian to ensure that the diet meets your nutritional needs. You may also wish to talk with your doctor about screening for other conditions; this is especially true for celiac disease, because a low-FODMAP plan can make screening inaccurate.

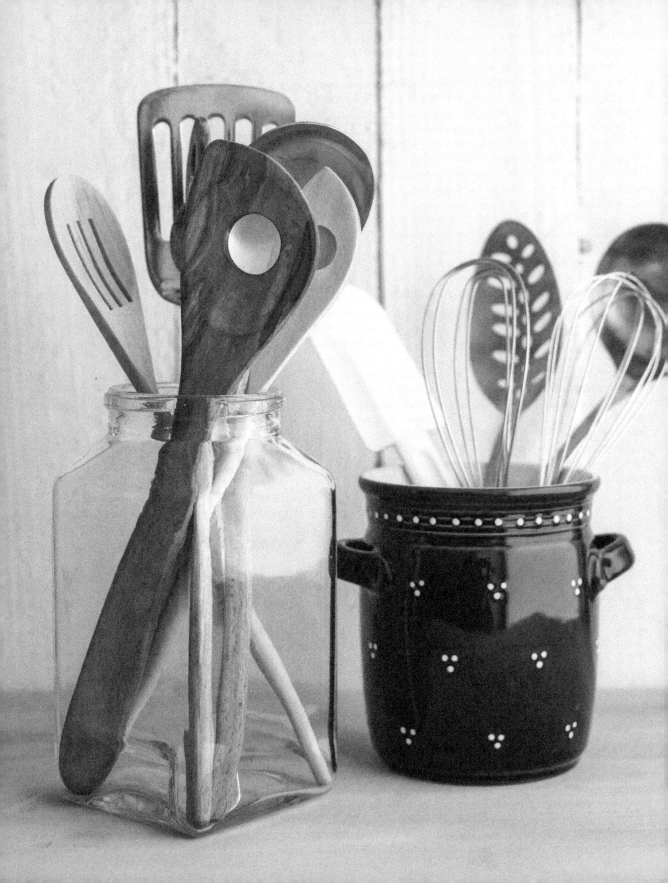

CONTENTS

INTRODUCTION

from LAURA

Many people with a healthy functioning gastrointestinal (GI) system take it for granted. When the digestive system works properly we experience few problems as we eat and digest our food. When we eat food, our bodies break it down and absorb the nutrients we need for life. But what happens when something goes wrong with this important system? It's not like we can stop eating and drinking to give our GI system a break.

As a registered dietitian practicing clinically, I am intimately familiar with the stresses people suffer from the IBS experience. The daily struggle with IBS symptoms can have a major effect on every aspect of my clients' existence—from their professional to their personal and social lives.

When people with IBS and other GI dysfunctions are unable to metabolize foods in a healthy or efficient manner, it can be helpful to make dietary changes—not only to what we eat, but also with regard to the structure and timing of meals. The low-FODMAP diet achieves this for people suffering from IBS, and there is a great deal of peer-reviewed scientific evidence confirming that it works. This diet is a *temporary* eating plan that can help you calm and quiet your digestive symptoms by eliminating foods that may be irritating your bowel. Then, after several weeks of calming the gut, you begin to reintroduce foods to identify what works for you and what you need to avoid.

As a dietitian, I have helped numerous patients through this process, and it is always a joy to witness how the low-FODMAP diet helps their symptoms abate as they learn what works best for them. They acquire the information they need to make informed choices about what foods to eat, and they regain a sense of power and control. The low-FODMAP diet and the variations you'll find in this book have given many of my clients their lives back, so they can return to the things that really matter to them, without having to worry about uncomfortable symptom flare-ups.

I am thrilled to share this diet with you. I wish you good health.

from KAREN

Hello, fellow GI-symptom sufferers. I completely understand how debilitating and life affecting gastrointestinal distress can be. Since my early twenties (I'm 50 now!) I've spent countless hours in doctors' offices seeking diagnoses for my gastrointestinal symptoms. I've had virtually every GI test imaginable, many featuring tubes and cameras, that were unpleasant, to say the least.

There were days when it was difficult to leave the house because I wasn't sure when I'd need to run to the bathroom. My stomach hurt constantly, and I was so tired of feeling bad. While my ultimate diagnosis was celiac disease (not, as had been tentatively diagnosed several times, IBS or IBD), just knowing what was wrong with me was a tremendous source of empowerment. Suddenly, I had the information I needed to regain my health and my life.

But then, there was the diet. When I looked at eliminating food groups—FODMAPs, with my first diagnosis, and then everything containing gluten with my final diagnosis—I was intimidated. These were foods I loved, and giving them up was daunting. I played with eliminating foods when I felt like it. I would think, "How bad could it really be?" and I'd ingest something I knew was harmful to me. Then I'd be right back where I started.

I finally got serious about sticking to the diet, and my health changed forever. During the years I sought diagnoses, I tried many restrictive diets. Quickly, I learned the best way to stick to an eating program was by cooking foods I enjoyed eating so much that I didn't miss the things I could no longer have. Now, I seek to empower others to heal their bodies through dietary means, offering delicious, easy-to-make, affordable recipes for people on specialized diets. It's my philosophy that there's no single "healthy" diet, but rather a nutritious diet that works for you.

The recipes in this book are designed to assist you in finding the diet that helps you manage your symptoms, with foods that are so satisfying and easy to prepare, you won't miss the ingredients you've eliminated.

The
LOW-
FODMAP
DIET

1

If you're looking at this low-FODMAP diet cookbook, chances are you've been diagnosed with (or strongly suspect you have) irritable bowel syndrome.

In the following chapters, we discuss IBS and the subtypes and related conditions of the disorder. You'll learn what a FODMAP is, and why that is important knowledge for you to have with your IBS diagnosis. You'll find a useful list of foods to avoid. You'll learn how to follow a temporary low-FODMAP diet for several weeks to help calm your symptoms and then how to reintroduce food items to discover which ones are your personal triggers. In this way, you can create a customized eating plan for life.

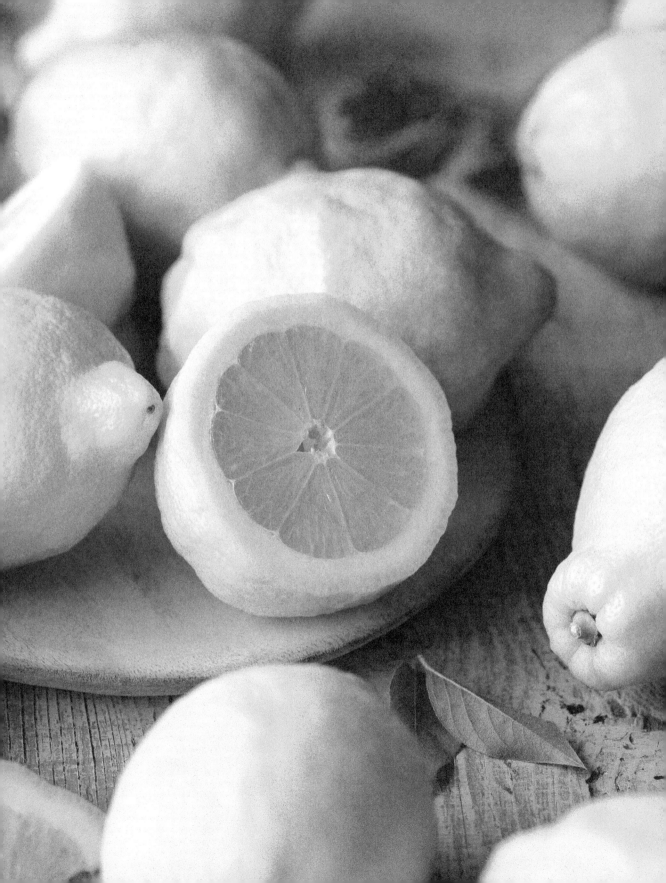

1

THE LOW-FODMAP DIET
FOR DIGESTIVE DISORDERS

If you're one of the 25 to 45 million people who suffer from irritable bowel syndrome, you know how frustrating and debilitating the condition can be. While no single diet works for all people, following a low-FODMAP diet for several weeks lets you create a particular eating plan that will control your symptoms. It takes some organization and effort on your part, as well as care in tracking your symptoms. But the time and effort spent will help you regain your quality of life.

Many people who have followed a low-FODMAP diet and identified and eliminated their own personal food triggers have noticed vast improvements in their general health. Condition flare-ups occur less frequently—or not at all! You can have the same experience.

This book offers help in the forms of practical advice, a customizable temporary diet to determine the best way for you to eat, and more than 100 tasty, nutritious recipes and 4 low-FODMAP meal plans. This book will help you stick to a temporary elimination diet to calm your gut. Then we will guide you, step by step, through the process of customization, helping you track symptoms as you reintroduce foods to discover which ones help keep your gut calm and which ones trigger symptoms. Ultimately, you'll wind up with a diet friendly for the type of IBS and the symptoms you have—a custom eating plan to remain as symptom-free as possible so you can live life to the fullest.

IBS TYPES & COEXISTING CONDITIONS

According to the International Foundation for Functional Gastrointestinal Disorders (IFFGD), about 10 to 15 percent of the world's population suffers from IBS. Women are more likely to be affected than men (about two-thirds of all sufferers are women), and it can affect people of any age.

The exact cause of IBS is unknown, although research is ongoing. The primary symptom of IBS is long-term and recurrent gastrointestinal (GI) discomfort and pain, which arises from impaired GI function. Also frequently present are bloating and gas. Symptoms can vary vastly from person to person, which often makes IBS tricky to diagnose and treat. Currently, experts have identified multiple types of IBS and coexisting conditions, including

- IBS-A (alternating constipation and diarrhea)
- IBS-C (constipation dominant)
- IBS-D (diarrhea dominant)
- IBS plus acid reflux (GERD)
- IBD plus IBS overlay
- IBS plus celiac disease
- IBS plus food allergies
- IBS plus small intestinal bacterial overgrowth (a less-common occurrence)

Conditions can coexist that may indicate certain dietary changes should be made outside of a typical low-FODMAP plan, and therefore many of the recipes in this book offer tips for changes to accommodate other health issues.

IBS-A

Also known as IBS-Alternating Type or simply IBS, IBS-A occurs when someone diagnosed with IBS has alternating bouts of constipation and diarrhea. People with this type of IBS may experience about a quarter of their stools as watery and consistent with diarrhea and about a quarter of their stools as hard and lumpy, consistent with constipation. These stool changes may occur regularly, or the person may go for several weeks or months with one type of stool and then switch to the other type for several weeks or months. This inconsistency in bowel habits makes this form difficult to diagnose and treat. All recipes included here are designed to help IBS-Alternating Type, but also can be modified for other types of IBS and conditions.

IBS-C

Constipation-dominant IBS (IBS-C) is perhaps the most commonly occurring form of the condition. People with IBS-C may experience pain with infrequent bowel movements, straining to pass stools, or hard, lumpy stools. The IFFGD notes that, on average, people with IBS-C report episodes of pain, gas, bloating, and constipation—with or without nausea—occurring more than 200 times per year.

IBS-D

People with IBS-D, or diarrhea-dominant IBS, experience frequent watery or loose stools with great urgency, accompanied by abdominal pain, cramping, and/or nausea, and an increased rate of bowel movements. Some also report loss of bowel control.

IBS PLUS ACID REFLUX

Acid reflux, or gastroesophageal reflux disease (GERD), is a condition that commonly occurs in conjunction with IBS-A, IBS-C, or IBS-D. While IBS occurs in the lower GI tract (stomach and intestines), acid reflux occurs in the upper GI region (stomach, lower esophageal sphincter [LES], and esophagus). Symptoms of IBS may be as discussed previously, while acid reflux often presents as burning in the stomach or throat, which results from acid washing up through the lower esophageal sphincter and into the throat.

A study published in the *World Journal of Gastroenterology* in March 2010 found a 64 percent prevalence of GERD in female patients with IBS as opposed to a 34 percent prevalence in patients without IBS. This finding suggests an overlap between the two conditions, which requires further study to establish why the co-occurrence exists.

INFLAMMATORY BOWEL DISEASE (IBD) PLUS IBS OVERLAY

IBD is an autoimmune disease of the bowel, such as Crohn's disease or colitis. Inflammatory diseases involve chronic inflammation of the GI tract. It's important to note that the two conditions are distinct from each other. In some cases, however, physicians find that people in remission from IBD may experience IBS symptoms. One study published in the October 2012 issue of the *American Journal of Gastroenterology* noted that in these patients, IBS presented with subtle inflammatory changes even though the inflammatory condition of IBD was in remission. This finding suggests there may be some inflammatory processes at play in IBS, particularly in the case of IBD with IBS overlay.

IBS PLUS CELIAC DISEASE

Celiac disease is a condition in which the body has an autoimmune response to the ingestion of gluten (protein substances in some cereal grains, like wheat). In celiac disease, even trace amounts of gluten cause damage to the villi (small fingerlike projections responsible for nutrient absorption) in the intestines, which creates pain, inflammation, and the inability to absorb nutrients from certain foods. Symptoms of celiac disease are very similar to those of IBS, and can include pain, bloating, gas, nausea, and diarrhea, among others. Since celiac disease is often initially misdiagnosed as IBS, it's important to seek blood test screening for antibodies and have your doctor obtain biopsies from your small intestine via an endoscopy *before* undertaking a low-FODMAP diet, since this diet can affect the outcome of the test. While the two conditions can occur together, it is important to rule out celiac disease before arriving at an IBS diagnosis.

IBS PLUS FOOD ALLERGIES

Food allergies occur when your body has an immune response to ingested substances. It's important to distinguish food allergies (immune response) from food sensitivities/intolerances, in which the body often has a GI response, because allergic responses can be life threatening (can lead to anaphylaxis), while sensitivities and intolerances will not. For example, someone who has a milk intolerance may have a GI response to the lactose in milk, creating gas, bloating, and loose stools, while someone with a milk allergy may have an immune system response (including inflammation) to the casein in dairy products. In either case, it's best to avoid these foods, and it's critical if you are allergic.

Both food sensitivities and allergies may play a role in IBS, although more studies are needed to understand this issue. Likewise, because food allergies and sensitivities are so commonplace, you may find you have both conditions occurring simultaneously. Therefore, it is important to adapt your dietary strategy so you avoid foods to which you are allergic or sensitive, even if they are allowable on your low-FODMAP diet. Otherwise, inflammation and GI irritation related to the food sensitivity or allergy may prevent you from experiencing relief in spite of dietary changes.

SMALL INTESTINAL BACTERIAL OVERGROWTH (SIBO)

SIBO is a condition in which the small intestine contains an unusually large number of bacteria that have migrated up from the colon. Symptoms of SIBO include abdominal distention, painful bloating with constipation/diarrhea, or both. The colon is typically where bacteria reside. In some instances such as post-infectious -IBS, IBD, untreated celiac disease, motility disorders of the gut, among others, the low-FODMAP diet may be helpful in modifying the bacterial load in your gut. Your doctor may want to conduct a breath test to establish whether you have bacterial overgrowth and potentially treat it with an antibiotic as well as recommend that the low-FODMAP diet be used post-treatment. The low-FODMAP diet may be an additional helpful tool to manage this painful and irritating condition.

RECENT IBS RESEARCH

Recent research suggests that our gut microbiome (the bacteria in our intestines) may play a role in GI conditions such as IBS. One article in the October 2014 issue of *World Journal of Gastroenterology* explored this relationship, concluding that the gut microbiome may play a role in both triggering and calming symptoms. This suggestion has led to increased interest in foods and substances that change the structure of the microbiome, such as fermented and cultured foods and probiotics. But because probiotics can worsen symptoms in a weakened digestive system, the recipes in this book do *not* include fermented foods.

UNDERSTANDING FODMAPS

So what is a FODMAP anyway, and why should you eliminate it from your diet?

FODMAPs, or *fermentable oligosaccharides, disaccharides, monosaccharides, and polyols*, are certain types of *carbohydrates* naturally occurring in foods that the small intestine absorbs poorly, although not everyone has an issue with FODMAPs. These short-chain carbohydrates, because they are poorly absorbed, travel to the small intestine where the bacteria use them for fuel. In some people this may lead to symptoms commonly associated with IBS, such as gas, bloating, and diarrhea. And so if you're sensitive to FODMAPs, you may experience symptoms of IBS when you ingest them.

Carbohydrates in the category FODMAPs include

- **Fructose:** A simple sugar found in honey and many fruits such as cherries, mango, and watermelon.
- **Lactose:** A simple sugar found in milk and dairy products.
- **Fructans:** Polymers of fructose found in certain grains such as wheat, as well as in onions and garlic.
- **Galactans:** Complex carbohydrates found in legumes such as kidney beans and black beans.

- **Polyols:** Sugar alcohols, such as maltitol, erythritol, and others, commonly found in sugar-free foods such as gums and low-calorie or diabetic-friendly foods.

Many people with IBS may be sensitive to FODMAPs, and so eliminating them from or minimizing them in your diet can help you avoid symptoms of poor absorption.

FOODS WITH FODMAPS

Since you don't want to guess at which foods contain high levels of FODMAPs, which ones might be okay to have in small amounts, and which ones you can eat freely, the following chart can help you determine the best ways to eat as you follow a FODMAP elimination diet. You can also find this information in a handy smartphone app, the Monash University Low-FODMAP Diet app.

THE LOW-FODMAP ELIMINATION DIET

The low-FODMAP diet is a *temporary* elimination diet that you will follow for 2 to 6 weeks to help calm your gut—and your symptoms. Once your symptoms have calmed and been absent, you can begin the reintroduction phase to identify which foods are your personal triggers.

To learn from this diet, it is important to track your symptoms throughout the duration. It's easy to forget how severe your symptoms were once they disappear, so use the tracker (page 26) to record symptoms *before*, *during*, and *after* the elimination and reintroduction phases of the diet.

LOW-FODMAP **FOODS TO ENJOY**	MODERATE-FODMAP **FOODS TO TASTE** (just a bit)	HIGH-FODMAP **FOODS TO AVOID**

Dairy

2 to 3 servings per day; **1 serving = ½ cup** Cheese: Brie, Camembert, Cheddar, feta, mozzarella, Parmesan, Swiss; Ice cream (lactose-free); Milk: almond, coconut (canned), lactose-free, rice; Yogurt: goat's milk, Greek-style, lactose-free	**Amount per day limited** **to those listed below** Butter (1 tablespoon); Cheese: cottage (2 tablespoons), ricotta (2 tablespoons); Half-and-half (1 tablespoon); Heavy (whipping) cream (1 tablespoon)	Buttermilk; Cream cheese; Custard; Halloumi (cheese); Ice cream; Milk: cow's, goat's, soy; Pudding; Sour cream; Yogurt

Fruit

2 to 3 servings per day; **1 serving = 1 medium piece** **or 1 cup diced** Banana (½), Blueberries, Breadfruit, Cantaloupe, Clementine, Dragon fruit, Durian, Grapes, Guava (ripe), Honeydew melon, Kiwi, Kumquat, Lemon, Lime, Mandarin orange, Orange, Passion fruit, Paw paw, Pineapple, Plantain, Prickly pear, Raspberries, Rhubarb, Star fruit, Strawberries, Tamarind	**Amount per day limited** **to those listed below** Avocado (¼), Coconut, fresh or flaked (½ cup)	Apple, Apricot, Blackberries, Boysenberries, Cherries, Figs, Grapefruit, Guava (unripened), Lychee, Mango, Nectarine, Peach, Pear, Persimmon, Plum, Pomegranate, Watermelon

LOW-FODMAP **FOODS TO ENJOY**	MODERATE-FODMAP **FOODS TO TASTE** (just a bit)	HIGH-FODMAP **FOODS TO AVOID**

Vegetables

5 to 7 servings per day; 1 = serving 1 cup raw or ½ cup cooked	**Amount per day limited to those listed below**	Artichokes: globe, Jerusalem; Asparagus; Beet; Cabbage, savoy; Cassava; Cauliflower; Corn, sweet; Garlic; Leek (white part only); Mushrooms; Onion; Peas; Shallots; Sweet potato; Taro root; Yucca
Arugula; Beans, green; Bean sprouts; Bell pepper: green, red; Bok choy; Broccoli; Brussels sprouts; Cabbage: green, red; Carrot; Celery root (celeriac); Chicory leaves; Chile pepper: green, red; Collard greens; Cucumber; Eggplant; Endive; Fennel; Kale; Leek (green part only); Lettuce; Okra; Olives; Parsnip; Pickles; Potato; Radicchio; Radish; Scallion (green part only); Seaweed; Spinach; Squash: spaghetti, summer, zucchini; Swiss chard; Tomato; Turnip	Artichoke hearts, canned (¼ cup); Butternut squash (½ cup); Celery (1 stalk); Pumpkin (1 cup)	

Legumes

Tempeh, 1 (3½-ounce) slice; Tofu, firm not silken (⅔ cup)	**Amount per day limited to those listed below**	Beans of all kinds except chickpeas and lentils
	Chickpeas, canned (¼ cup); Lentils (canned, scant ½ cup)	

LOW-FODMAP **FOODS TO ENJOY**	MODERATE-FODMAP **FOODS TO TASTE** (just a bit)	HIGH-FODMAP **FOODS TO AVOID**

Grains & Cereals

At least 4 servings per day; 1 serving = 2 slices bread, 2 corn tortillas, ⅔ cup flour, 1 cup cereal, 1 cup cooked whole grains Buckwheat; Corn tortillas; Gluten-free bread, cereal, pasta, etc. (made without added honey or agave); Millet; Oats, gluten-free; Quinoa; Rice; Starch, potato; Tapioca	**Amount per day limited to those listed below** Corn flakes (½ cup); Oatmeal: uncooked, not gluten-free (½ cup); uncooked, quick cooking (¼ cup); Puffed rice cereal (½ cup)	Amaranth; Barley; Bread: multi-grain, rye, wheat; Couscous; Einkorn; Emmer; Granola; Muesli; Pasta, wheat; Rice Krispies; Rye; Spelt; Wheat; Wheat bran

Nuts & Seeds

2 tablespoons seeds per day; 1 small handful nuts per day Brazil nuts; Chestnuts; Chia seeds; Macadamia nuts; Peanuts; Pecans; Pine nuts; Poppy seeds; Pumpkin seeds (shelled); Sesame seeds; Sunflower seeds (shelled); Walnuts	**Amount per day limited to those listed below** Hazelnuts (10)	Cashews; Pistachios

LOW-FODMAP **FOODS TO ENJOY**	MODERATE-FODMAP **FOODS TO TASTE** (just a bit)	HIGH-FODMAP **FOODS TO AVOID**

Herbs, Spices & Flavorings

Enjoy unlimited amounts Allspice, Basil, Bay leaf, Caraway, Cardamom, Chives, Cilantro/coriander, Cinnamon, Cloves, Cumin, Curry, Dill, Garlic oil, Ginger, Marjoram, Mint, Mustard, Nutmeg, Oregano, Paprika, Parsley, Rosemary, Sage, Thyme, Vanilla		Chicory root (inulin), Garlic powder, Onion powder

Sweeteners

Limit to 1 serving per day Stevia (2 packets); Sugar: brown, white (1 tablespoon); Syrup, pure maple (2 tablespoons)		Agave; Honey; Sugar alcohols

Condiments

Capers; Chutney; Horseradish; Mayonnaise, homemade; Paste: miso, tamarind, tomato; Sauce: fish, oyster, soy, Worcestershire; Tahini (sesame seed paste 1 tablespoon); Vinegar: apple cider, red wine, rice, white	**Amount per day limited to those listed below** Hummus, made without garlic (¼ cup); Pesto, made without garlic (1 tablespoon); Vinegar, balsamic (2 tablespoons)	Ketchup, Relish, Tzatziki

LOW-FODMAP **FOODS TO ENJOY**	MODERATE-FODMAP **FOODS TO TASTE** (just a bit)	HIGH-FODMAP **FOODS TO AVOID**

Meat, Poultry, Eggs & Seafood

1 to 2 servings per day; **1 serving = 3 ounces** Any		

Fats & Oils

	In moderate amounts; **4 tablespoons per day** Oil: canola, coconut, olive, vegetable	

Other

Chocolate, dark (2 [1-ounce] squares)	**Amount per day limited** **to those listed below** Chocolate: milk (1 ounce); white (1 ounce)	

PHASE 1: ELIMINATION

During the elimination phase, you will

- eliminate all high-FODMAP foods (see chart, pages 18–22) from your diet,
- strictly limit moderate-FODMAP foods to the amounts listed in the chart, and
- enjoy any foods listed as low-FODMAP foods in the chart.

Steps to implement this elimination phase:

a. Talk with your doctor before you begin this diet.

b. Track your symptoms for a few days before starting.

c. Plan to remain in the elimination phase for a minimum of 2 weeks. If symptoms persist after 2 weeks, continue for 2 weeks more, or as needed until you feel about 80 percent better than when you started.

d. If after 6 weeks you remain symptomatic, it is important to talk to your doctor again to rule out other conditions.

e. Determine which type of IBS you have (IBS-A, IBS-C, or IBS-D, as well as any coexisting conditions). Choose the meal plan that works best for your IBS type (see pages 14–16), and follow any recipe tips to help eliminate other foods as necessary for coexisting conditions.

f. Begin the diet, following it as outlined in the meal plan. You may make substitutions from other recipes in this book using the provided tips to adapt to your individual needs.

g. As you follow the diet, continue to track symptoms.

SAMPLE FOODS

Containing One Individual FODMAP Suitable for Challenging Tolerance Levels

All of the foods in this list can take up to 3 days to test.

FODMAP	CHALLENGE FOOD
Polyol (sorbitol)	Avocado
Galactan	Chickpeas
Fructan	Garlic
note that within this category, garlic, wheat, and onions should be tested separately	
Fructose	Honey
Fructan	Onion
Lactose	Milk
Fructan	Persimmon
Polyol (mannitol)	Sweet potato
Fructan	Wheat bread
Fructan	Wheat pasta

PHASE 2: REINTRODUCTION

During Phase 2 of the diet, you will reintroduce foods by category (chemical component): fructose, lactose, fructans, galactans, and polyols. This procedure will allow you to customize the diet for your individual needs. The chart offers some sample foods for each FODMAP to use for testing during this phase; all of the foods in this list can take up to 3 days to test. Also review Understanding FODMAPs, page 17.

To reintroduce foods:

a. Reintroduce a single food at a time while remaining on the low-FODMAP diet. For example, if you wish to start with lactose, complete the following steps:

- Choose one high-lactose dairy food such as milk or yogurt.

- Eat a small amount (½ cup) with a meal.

- Consume this food once a day in the same small portion for 3 days.

- Continue to track your symptoms.

b. If you have symptoms, this is a food you will not be able to eat in large quantities because it makes you symptomatic. Track your symptoms, and put it aside for a while. You may be able to reintroduce it again at a later date in a smaller quantity.

c. If you don't have symptoms after the 3-day test period, for the next 2 days increase the amount of the food you consume by 1½ to 2 times. Track your symptoms and listen to your body. Everyone's tolerance varies.

d. If you remain asymptomatic, you have passed the test for this category and can begin a new one. Record your lack of symptoms.

e. If symptoms recur, discontinue the food and put it on your "limit" list. Give yourself a 3-day break by returning to the low-FODMAP diet as you did in the elimination phase.

f. Be sure to return to the low-FODMAP diet and eliminate the lactose food, or other item you are testing, while you reintroduce the next food.

g. After a week of testing foods within a food group (chemical component), move on to another group (for instance, fructans, testing onions and garlic.)

h. *Only introduce one food group at a time, tracking symptoms as you do, and discontinuing foods that make you symptomatic.*

PHASE 3: LIFETIME EATING

Once you've reintroduced all foods, you will know which foods will make up your lifetime eating plan to help you remain symptom-free. Avoid any foods that cause symptoms. If you experience a flare-up, return to 1 to 2 weeks of strict low-FODMAP eating to quiet your gut. There's no need to go through reintroduction again unless you suspect you've developed new intolerances.

MEAL PLANS FOR SPECIFIC CONDITIONS/ SYMPTOMS

The meal plans in this book are designed so you can switch from plan to plan, if necessary, depending on other conditions and symptoms. For example, you may do 2 weeks of IBS-C and then switch to Acid Reflux if you have that condition. It is important to listen to your body as you follow this diet.

TRACKING YOUR SYMPTOMS

The most important time to track symptoms is during reintroduction of FODMAP foods. It is essential to introduce only one FODMAP at a time or you won't know which foods cause symptoms. You can do this for FODMAP *groups* instead of single foods, since it is typically a group of FODMAPs you react to rather than a single food. Let's take a look at the groups and some of the foods that fall in those groups.

FRUCTOSE

Foods that contain high amounts of fructose:

- Foods made with high fructose corn syrup
- Fruits and dried fruits such as mango, watermelon, and cherries
- Fruit juices
- Honey
- Ketchup
- Processed fruits (canned, jarred, frozen; processed with sugar)

LACTOSE

Foods that contain high amounts of lactose:

- Ice cream
- Kefir
- Milk
- Soft cheese
- Sour cream
- Yogurt

FRUCTANS

Foods that contain high amounts of fructans:

- Artichokes
- Barley
- Beets
- Garlic
- Grapefruit
- Inulin/chicory root
- Leek
- Onion
- Peas
- Pomegranate
- Rye
- Spelt
- Stone fruits
- Wheat
- Watermelon

GALACTANS

Foods containing high amounts of galactans include:

- Certain types of cabbage
- Legumes
- Soy

POLYOLS

Foods containing high amounts of polyols:

- Stone fruits
- Sugar-free medicines, gums, and candies
- Sugar alcohols

Symptom Tracker

Use this page to track symptoms. Make as many copies as you need so you can continue to track symptoms as you reintroduce foods.

DATE	FOOD REINTRODUCED	AMOUNT	SYMPTOMS	DESIGNATION (OKAY, LIMIT, AVOID)

It's important to note that some foods contain more than one type of FODMAP. This is where you will find the Monash Low-FODMAP app handy. It can help you know exactly what type of FODMAPs each food contains so you can introduce each one appropriately during the reintroduction phase. For example, if a food falls into two groups, you should test each component separately. If you experience symptoms from either component, then avoid that food.

PREPARING YOUR KITCHEN AND PANTRY

Since we are working to eliminate foods that cause symptoms, you'll be making most of your meals from scratch using whole, natural foods. While the recipes here are quick and simple, having the following staples on hand will be helpful.

FATS AND OILS

You'll primarily use extra-virgin olive oil. However, if you have another oil preference, you can use that. You will also make Garlic Oil (page 184), which can be stored in a clean container in your pantry, to add flavor to the foods you eat.

CONDIMENTS, HERBS, AND SPICES

You'll want the following condiments, herbs, and spices on hand:

- Barbecue Sauce, homemade (page 180)
- Dijon mustard
- Dried herbs such as oregano, rosemary, sage, tarragon, and thyme
- Ground spices such as allspice, black pepper, cinnamon, coriander, cumin, curry powder, nutmeg, and sea salt
- Vinegar: apple cider, red wine, white

OTHER SHELF-STABLE ITEMS

Keeping a well-stocked pantry means fewer trips to the grocery store, so keep some of the following shelf-stable items handy:

- Arrowroot powder
- Baking powder, gluten-free
- Bread, gluten-free, wheat-free (such as UDI's sandwich bread, which is also low in FODMAPs)
- Chickpeas, canned
- Corn tortillas
- Dark chocolate, unsweetened
- Dark cocoa powder, unsweetened
- Flour, gluten-free, wheat-free (King Arthur gluten-free flour is an excellent blend because it is also low in FODMAPs)
- Lentils, canned
- Mayonnaise, homemade (page 178)
- Milk: coconut (canned) and rice
- Miso paste
- Oil: olive (extra-virgin) and coconut
- Peanut butter (sugar-free)
- Rice: brown and white
- Sauce: fish, soy (gluten-free or regular), Worcestershire

- Stevia
- Sugar: brown and white
- Sunflower seeds (shelled)
- Tomatoes, canned
- Tomato paste
- Tomato sauce (made without garlic and onions)

ESSENTIAL KITCHEN EQUIPMENT

You likely have some of the equipment listed here. If not, you may find some of the following items convenient to have on hand:

- Baking pans (9-by-13-inch; 9-by-9-inch; and 9-by-5-inch loaf pans)
- Baking sheets
- Blender and/or food processor
- Citrus zester or rasp-style grater
- Cutting board that is never used to cut conventional bread or other gluten-containing ingredients
- Large Dutch oven with a lid that can go from stove top to oven, for making soups and stews
- Large skillet or sauté pan
- Parchment paper and aluminum foil
- Sharp knives, including a chef's knife and paring knife
- Spiral vegetable cutter, a mandoline, or a julienne peeler

LOW-FODMAP INGREDIENTS AND FOOD ALLERGEN SUBSTITUTIONS

Depending on your food allergies or sensitivities, you'll want some staples on hand before you get started with your diet.

- **Garlic Oil (page 184):** Flavorful and easy to make by simmering garlic cloves in olive oil.
- **Sunflower Butter (page 187):** If you're allergic to peanuts, replace peanut butter with sunflower butter. Store, refrigerated and tightly sealed, for up to 1 month.
- **If you're allergic to eggs,** make a flaxseed egg substitute low in FODMAPs. For each egg called for in a recipe, combine 1 tablespoon ground flaxseed with 3 tablespoons water. Mix well and refrigerate for 15 minutes. You can also use ground chia seeds in the same ratio.

- Storage containers with lids (refrigerator- and freezer-safe) for homemade condiments, leftovers, etc.
- Wooden spoons that are never used to mix gluten-containing ingredients

FOR MODIFIED TEXTURES

Some of the food plans in the book require modified textures, which can be helpful for people with IBD/IBS-D because they are gentler on the stomach and easier to digest. To modify the texture of your foods, you will need one of the following:

Food Allergen Substitutions

COMMON ALLERGEN	SUBSTITUTION	NOTES
Eggs	Flaxseed or chia seed eggs (see sidebar on page 28); tofu (for scrambled eggs)	Flaxseed or chia seed eggs work for baking. Tofu works for scrambled eggs (if you're not allergic to soy).
Peanuts	Macadamia nuts Macadamia butter or sunflower butter	Finely chop the nuts; use a 1:1 substitution.
Tree nuts	Sunflower seeds (shelled) Pepitas (shelled pumpkin seeds)	Shelled sunflower seeds or pumpkin seeds (pepitas) add the crunch you get from nuts.
Milk, lactose-free	Rice or hemp milk, coconut milk (canned)	Use a 1:1 substitution. Choose unsweetened, plain.
Fish	Shellfish or poultry	Use an equal amount of shellfish or white meat poultry in place of fish in recipes.
Shellfish	White fish or poultry	Use an equal amount of white fish or white meat poultry in place of shellfish in recipes.
Yogurt, lactose-free	Coconut yogurt	Choose plain, unsweetened, no fruit added. Add your own low-FODMAP fruit.
Soy sauce	Worcestershire sauce or fish sauce	Substitute Worcestershire sauce at a 1:1 ratio. Substitute fish sauce at a ½:1 ratio.
Cheese	Hemp cheese Nutritional yeast	Hemp cheese grates like regular cheese and can be substituted at a 1:1 ratio. Nutritional yeast works well to replace grated Parmesan or Asiago cheese for sprinkling.

- Blender, regular or immersion
- Food mill
- Food processor

If you already have one or more of these, you're in good shape. Otherwise, choose one that will work best for your needs and budget.

SETTING YOURSELF UP FOR SUCCESS

Any time you go on a restrictive diet, temptation can get in the way. No one likes to feel deprived. There are steps, however, you can take to set yourself up for success as you follow the low-FODMAP diet.

Always track your symptoms. Keeping track of how much better you feel is quite motivating, and looking back at how badly you once felt can help keep you from backsliding or thinking that, just this once, a little dab of something your body reacts to won't hurt.

Prepare ahead of time. Clear your cupboards, refrigerator, and pantry of items that will tempt you. Get rid of that jar of honey and the wheat bread. Instead, stock up on foods you know will support your body as you progress toward healing.

Enlist support. Let your friends and family know what you are doing and why you are doing it. Ask that they support you in this, explaining it is of utmost importance for your health and well-being. If you inform people ahead of time, they will be less likely to tempt you with a little bite of this or that, which may cause your symptoms to reoccur.

Cook ahead whenever you can. Because you will be making most of your meals from scratch, cooking ahead is a great way to stay on track. On the weekends, prepare meals ahead of time and refrigerate or freeze them for the coming week.

Double or triple a batch for leftovers. Moving forward after the initial meal plan, making large batches and eating leftovers saves tons of time. Cooking once and eating twice, or more, is a huge time-saver (and stress reliever). Take leftovers for lunches or cook enough to get at least two dinners out of every recipe.

Make stocks and sauces in large batches and freeze them. This is where freezer containers come in handy. You can make stock, ketchup, and other sauces ahead of time and freeze them in individual servings or weekly batches. They'll be ready whenever you need them.

Chop fresh herbs ahead of time and freeze them. Fill ice cube trays with 1 tablespoon of chopped fresh herbs and top them with 1 tablespoon of olive oil. Freeze and then store them in labeled freezer bags. Whenever you need to add herbs to something, pop out a cube and toss it in whatever you're cooking.

Focus on what you *can* have, not on what you can't. While the diet may feel restrictive in terms of all the things you can't eat, instead focus on all the wonderful foods you can enjoy. You'll be less likely to feel deprived. This simple mind shift can go a long way in helping you stay on track and feel satisfied.

Serve your family the same food you eat. One of the biggest pressures on time when you're on a special diet is cooking one thing for yourself and another thing for your family. These foods are designed to be tasty and family friendly, so you can cook one food for everyone to enjoy. If you wish, add an additional side dish for family members, but there is really no need to cook separate meals for everyone.

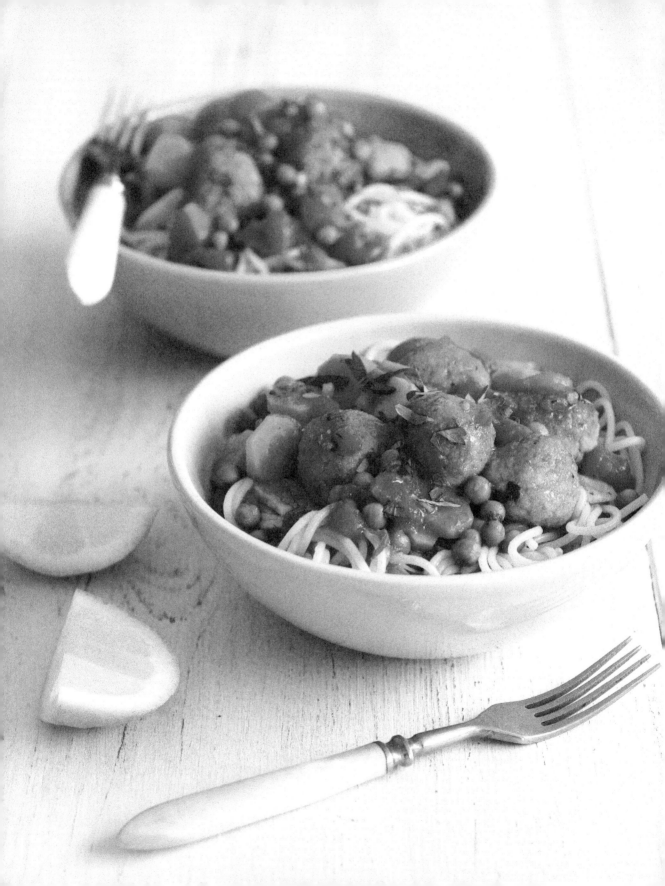

2

FLEXIBLE LOW-FODMAP
MEAL PLANS

Because IBS often occurs in conjunction with other GI issues, it's important for the plan to be flexible so you can eat in a way that best fits your unique health picture. That's why there are four different meal plans—you select the plan (or mix and match) that works best for where your health is right now. As you progress, you may find you need to switch to a different meal plan based on your current symptoms, which is okay. If you have IBS-A, then you may want to choose between the IBS-C and IBS-D plans depending on whether you are constipated or have diarrhea. If both constipation and diarrhea have resolved, you can follow the basic IBS plan. Likewise, you can use the tips included with each recipe to modify any recipe for your version of the plan.

The
BASIC LOW-FODMAP
MEAL PLAN

This meal plan is for people who have IBS without a specific type, or without other health challenges. The rules and principles of the plan are true for all plans within this cookbook, and all of the recipes in the book will be appropriate for a basic low-FODMAP diet.

EAT REGULAR MEALS

Now is *not* the time to skip meals. Because you are following an elimination diet, one of the best ways to stay psychologically prepared to stick with it is to avoid hunger. Therefore, make sure you eat regular meals: breakfast, lunch, dinner, and a snack or two. There's no need to feel deprived or hungry. If you are hungry, eat. This diet is about finding your way back to health, not about weight loss.

DO YOUR BEST NOT TO CHEAT

Temptation is natural when you're eliminating foods you enjoy, but to give your stomach and intestines the best help possible, it's important to stick with the foods on the list in chapter 1. Eating high-FODMAP foods, even in small amounts, can keep you from truly experiencing the benefits of this elimination diet, because they can keep symptoms active and mask other symptoms that can tell you certain foods aren't for you.

DON'T STAY ON THE ELIMINATION DIET INDEFINITELY

After 2 to 6 weeks, your symptoms will likely be much better. It's easy to get into the "diet" mentality of remaining strict to avoid discomfort. But the restrictive nature of the low-FODMAP elimination diet is intended to be temporary and may get tedious after a while; you'll want more variety. That's why it's important to eventually reintroduce foods and find the foods you can eat, so you have variety and create a diet sustainable for a lifetime.

REINTRODUCE FOODS ONE CATEGORY AT A TIME

The goal of a slow reintroduction schedule is to help you truly understand which foods cause symptoms and which don't. There is no one-size-fits-all diet here; it's important to understand that the diet is about discovering what works for you. After a period of being symptom-free, it's likely you'll know pretty quickly which types of FODMAPs cause symptoms in your body. These are the foods to eliminate for a lifetime.

MODIFY AS NEEDED

All the recipes in the book include modifications in texture and ingredients to fit various low-FODMAP plans, depending on your needs that day or that week. If you're experiencing diarrhea, choose the IBD/IBS-D option for that day to be gentle on your tummy. If you've noticed flare-ups of GERD, then try the GERD option instead.

MAKE SUBSTITUTIONS

It's okay to substitute one recipe for another, provided it fits your personal needs. For example, if there's a fish dish listed in the meal plan and you either don't like fish or are allergic to fish, then find another recipe to use in its place. Eating foods you enjoy and that make you feel well will go a long way toward making this way of eating sustainable. Likewise, within recipes you can make substitutions within reason—for example, substituting poultry for meat. However, don't substitute foods that are high in FODMAPs. *It's important that you avoid those until the reintroduction phase,* and then reintroduce them as recommended (see page 23).

DON'T FORGET FLUIDS

Drink plenty of fluids throughout this whole process. Staying hydrated will help you feel your best. Avoid soda, which contains high fructose corn syrup, and large amounts of juice (4 ounces max per day), which are concentrated sources of fructose. Instead, enjoy water, coffee, and tea (unless you have GERD and find that coffee and tea aggravate your condition). Wine and spirits are okay in moderate amounts, but realize that beer contains gluten and often wheat, while mixed drinks are often made with fructose-containing mixers. People with GERD may find consumption of any alcohol causes flare-ups, so it's best to avoid it in that case.

POSSIBLE CHALLENGES

Because of its restrictive nature, following an elimination diet can be challenging, particularly in the early stages as you get used to the "rules." Awareness of potential challenges can help you stay on track. It is best to be organized and prepared to prevent any additional stress.

CRAVINGS

Ah, cravings. It seems they are part of any elimination diet. It's natural to wish you could consume things that are suddenly off-limits. Be aware you may experience cravings, although these usually lessen as the diet progresses. Instead of focusing on what you can't have, focus on all the delicious foods you can eat and how much better you will feel when you identify your triggers. Keep healthy snacks on hand (from the foods-to-enjoy list, see pages 18–22, and chapter 5) to eat when you have a craving, and eat regularly so you don't get super hungry.

BOREDOM

When you're on a restrictive diet, it's easy to get bored with the foods you have available. Keep a wide variety of low-FODMAP foods handy, and avail yourself of a wide range of foods to help combat boredom and keep you on track.

CHANGING SYMPTOMS

You may notice that your symptoms change as you progress. For example, you may start out with IBS-D, but notice that constipation now seems to be your main symptom. To combat this, it's okay to switch plans and move to the plan that suits your current symptoms. Since all recipes are low in FODMAPs, you can find one that meets your needs at the moment.

SLIPUPS

We all slip up from time to time, especially when on a restrictive diet. If you do slip up, don't berate yourself. Instead, jump right back on the plan, drink plenty of fluids, and track any symptoms that arise.

DINING OUT

Dining out can be a bit tricky, as can going to someone else's house for dinner, or attending a party. If it's a party, bring low-FODMAP snacks for yourself and to share with others. If you're going to a friend's house, tell her about your low-FODMAP diet and offer to bring something to contribute to the menu. Or invite your friends to your home instead. In any instance eat only foods you know won't cause digestive issues.

If you're going out to dinner, review the menu ahead of time for low-FODMAP options. Don't go at peak hours, and talk to your server. I find that what works best for me in restaurants to make sure I don't get ingredients that cause me harm is to say I have an "allergy." Although, technically, you don't, servers and chefs take the word seriously.

FOUR WEEKS TO CONTROL IBS

Following is a 28-day meal plan for basic IBS, listing recipes found in the book. (Note that the listed food items that are initial capped are recipes in the book.) Remember to include one or two healthy snacks per day to control hunger. Shopping lists can be found on page 27.

WEEK ONE

MONDAY

Breakfast: Ginger Melon Smoothie, page 64

Lunch: Potato Leek Soup, page 84

Dinner: Spaghetti and Meatballs, page 146

TUESDAY

Breakfast: Maple-Cinnamon Oatmeal, page 66

Lunch: Turkey sandwich on Udi's gluten-free sandwich bread with 1 teaspoon Dijon mustard

Dinner: Veggie-Stuffed Trout, page 122

WEDNESDAY

Breakfast: PB&J Smoothie, page 62

Lunch: Kale Salad with Feta Cheese and Walnuts, page 88

Dinner: Pork Chops with Rhubarb Sauce, page 143

THURSDAY

Breakfast: Piña Colada Smoothie, page 61

Lunch: Tuna salad sandwich on Udi's gluten-free sandwich bread, made with 1 tablespoon Mayonnaise, page 178, mixed with 3 ounces water-packed tuna, drained

Dinner: Orange Chicken and Veggie Stir-Fry, page 140, and steamed rice

FRIDAY

Breakfast: Zucchini, Red Pepper, and Egg Scramble, page 73

Lunch: Easy Tomato Soup, page 78, with a grilled Cheddar cheese sandwich on Udi's gluten-free sandwich bread

Dinner: Pork Tenderloin with Asian Slaw, page 142

SATURDAY

Breakfast: Potato Hash with Fried Egg, page 72

Lunch: Shrimp Fried Rice, page 116

Dinner: Zucchini Lasagna, page 152

SUNDAY

Breakfast: Blueberry Pancakes, page 67

Lunch: Ground Turkey Stir-Fry, page 137

Dinner: Fish Curry, page 133

SNACKS FOR THE WEEK

Baked Green Bean "Fries," page 102

Zucchini Hummus (¼ cup per day max), page 101

Yogurt with Flaxseed and Blueberries, page 104

Sweet and Spicy Pecans, page 98

Sesame Kale Chips, page 100

WEEK TWO

MONDAY

Breakfast: Orange Chia Smoothie, page 63

Lunch: Egg salad sandwich: chop 2 hardboiled eggs, and mix in ½ grated carrot, 1 tablespoon Mayonnaise, page 178, and 1 teaspoon Dijon mustard, and serve on Udi's gluten-free sandwich bread

Dinner: Shrimp Scampi with Zucchini Noodles, page 117

TUESDAY

Breakfast: Lemon Dutch Baby, page 68

Lunch: Ground Beef and Veggie Soup, page 86

Dinner: Turkey Piccata, page 136, with steamed rice and veggies

WEDNESDAY

Breakfast: Dark Chocolate and Banana Smoothie, page 60

Lunch: Purchased rotisserie chicken with Potato Salad, page 93

Dinner: Maple-Soy Glazed Salmon with Tri-Pepper Sauté, page 126

THURSDAY

Breakfast: Bacon and Potato Frittata, page 70

Lunch: Baked potato with 1 tablespoon butter (or butter substitute), 1 ounce grated cheese, and shredded rotisserie chicken

Dinner: Minestrone, page 83

FRIDAY

Breakfast: Maple-Cinnamon Oatmeal, page 66

Lunch: Chopped Salad with Basil Vinaigrette, page 90

Dinner: Purchased rotisserie chicken with Warm Spinach Salad, page 89

SATURDAY

Breakfast: Ham Strata, page 75

Lunch: Clam Chowder, page 80

Dinner: Halibut with Rice and Pineapple Salsa, page 130

SUNDAY

Breakfast: Spiced Orange French Toast, page 69

Lunch: Broiled fish and Cucumber Salad with Asian Ginger Vinaigrette, page 91

Dinner: Hearty Meatloaf, page 144, with Loaded Smashed Potatoes, page 110

SNACKS FOR THE WEEK

Deviled Eggs, page 97

Baked Zucchini Chips, page 105

Spiced Roasted Pepitas, page 96

Chips and Salsa, page 109

Blueberry Muffins, page 106

WEEK THREE

MONDAY

Breakfast: 2 slices toast, made with Udi's gluten-free sandwich bread, spread with ¼ avocado

Lunch: Peanut butter (or Sunflower Butter, page 187) and half a banana sandwich on Udi's gluten-free sandwich bread

Dinner: Savory Vegetable Soup, page 79

TUESDAY

Breakfast: Blueberry Pancakes, page 67

Lunch: Chicken Soup with Zucchini Noodles, page 82

Dinner: Beef Fajitas, page 148

WEDNESDAY

Breakfast: Bell Pepper Omelet, page 74

Lunch: 2 slices Udi's gluten-free sandwich bread spread with Zucchini Hummus (¼ cup per day max), page 101, and topped with sliced cucumbers

Dinner: Shrimp and Grits, page 114

THURSDAY

Breakfast: Orange Chia Smoothie, page 63

Lunch: Simple Crab Salad, page 120

Dinner: Arroz con Pollo, page 141

FRIDAY

Breakfast: Spiced Orange French Toast, page 69

Lunch: Chef's salad made with iceberg lettuce, chopped turkey, 6 cherry tomatoes, and 1 carrot dressed with 2 tablespoons Basil Vinaigrette, page 185

Dinner: Bistro Burgers, page 150

SATURDAY

Breakfast: Bacon and Potato Frittata, page 70

Lunch: Fish and Chips, page 129

Dinner: Cottage Pie, page 154

SUNDAY

Breakfast: Lemon Dutch Baby, page 68

Lunch: Baked Mediterranean Turkey Meatballs with Roasted Red Pepper Sauce, page 151

Dinner: Pan-Seared Scallops with Orange Aioli, page 124

SNACKS FOR THE WEEK

Maple Corn Bread, page 111

Baked Potato Chips, page 99

Zucchini Hummus (¼ cup per day max), page 101

Hardboiled eggs

Spiced Roasted Pepitas, page 96

WEEK FOUR

MONDAY
Breakfast: Maple-Cinnamon Oatmeal, page 66

Lunch: Ground Beef and Veggie Soup, page 86

Dinner: Turkey Meatballs with Gingered Bok Choy, page 138

TUESDAY
Breakfast: Ginger Melon Smoothie, page 64

Lunch: Broiled chicken breast with Roasted Vegetable Salad, page 92

Dinner: Spaghetti and Meatballs, page 146

WEDNESDAY
Breakfast: Blueberry Muffins, page 106

Lunch: Roast beef sandwich on Udi's gluten-free sandwich bread with 2 tablespoons Mayonnaise, page 178, and 1 teaspoon prepared horseradish

Dinner: Cinnamon Shrimp, page 132

THURSDAY
Breakfast: Zucchini, Red Pepper, and Egg Scramble, page 73

Lunch: Easy Tomato Soup, page 78, and Maple Corn Bread, page 111

Dinner: Lemon Pepper Cod with Roasted Root Veggies, page 118

FRIDAY
Breakfast: Leftover Blueberry Muffins

Lunch: 2 hardboiled eggs and carrot sticks

Dinner: Orange Chicken and Veggie Stir-Fry, page 140

SATURDAY
Breakfast: Potato Hash with Fried Egg, page 72

Lunch: Hearty Fish Stew, page 128

Dinner: Zucchini Lasagna, page 152

SUNDAY
Breakfast: Lemon Dutch Baby, page 68

Lunch: Bistro Burgers, page 150

Dinner: Steamer Clams with Fennel in Broth, page 121, and Ambrosia Salad, page 87

SNACKS FOR THE WEEK
Chips and Salsa, page 109

Blueberry Muffins, page 106

Sesame Kale Chips, page 100

Sweet and Spicy Pecans, page 98

Yogurt with Flaxseed and Blueberries, page 104

The
LOW-FODMAP
MEAL PLAN FOR ACID REFLUX

Acid reflux presents its own unique challenges with unique requirements separate from a low-FODMAP diet. Therefore, if you suffer from GERD or regular acid reflux, this plan may be best for you. Follow these guidelines for managing acid reflux. Recipes appropriate for managing GERD or acid reflux (or that can be modified to be appropriate by following the "for Plan A" recipe tip) will be designated with an "A" icon.

EAT SEVERAL SMALL MEALS AND SNACKS

Overfilling your stomach can cause reflux by increasing abdominal pressure, which forces acid through the lower esophageal sphincter into the esophagus. Therefore, it is essential to eat several smaller meals instead of three large meals. You'll note in the recipes that the GERD guidelines suggest breaking up one serving into two and eating the servings 2 to 3 hours apart.

AVOID ACIDIC FOODS

Foods that are high in acid can cause flare-ups of acid reflux. To prevent these, avoid the following foods:

- Citrus juice
- Coffee
- Tomatoes
- Vinegar

AVOID OTHER FOOD TRIGGERS FOR GERD

There are other food triggers for GERD, including the following:

- Alcohol
- Bell peppers
- Caffeine
- Carbonated beverages
- Chile peppers
- Chocolate
- Garlic
- Onions
- Peppermint
- Spicy foods

AVOID HIGH-FAT FOODS

Foods that are high in fat can also trigger acid reflux, so it's important to minimize consumption of these added fat and fatty foods:

- Avocados
- Butter
- Fats and oils

- Fatty meats
- Fried foods
- Full-fat cheese
- Heavy (whipping) cream
- Mayonnaise

With these additional restrictions, recipes (when possible) have been adjusted for GERD.

POSSIBLE CHALLENGES

With a diet intended to address GERD symptoms, some of the following challenges may arise.

BLAND FOODS

Sometimes food on a GERD diet can seem particularly bland, because spice-laden foods often irritate the condition. Avoid black pepper, chili powder, paprika, and other chile pepper–based foods. Instead, use herbs and spices liberally as well as some vegetables to add flavor:

- Salt
- Ground sweet spices such as allspice, cinnamon, cloves, ginger, and nutmeg
- Ground savory spices such as cumin, coriander, mace, and turmeric
- Dried or fresh herbs such as basil, oregano, rosemary, sage, tarragon, and thyme
- Aromatic vegetables such as carrots and fennel

WHAT THE HECK DO YOU PUT ON A SALAD?

Because vinegars and citrus juices cause issues with GERD, and full-fat dressings may also be a problem, how do you dress a salad while managing for acid reflux? Use low-fat mayonnaise-based dressings, or low-fat lactose-free plain yogurt as a base, and mix in herbs, spices, and sea salt.

HUNGER

Some people feel like they're never quite satisfied with the small meal sizes that help them prevent GERD. Eating small amounts about 2 hours apart can keep you from getting hungry; if you feel yourself getting hungry, eat something—but just a little bit.

ACID REFLUX IS TRIGGERED ANYWAY

In some cases, acid reflux persists. If this is the case for you,

- talk with your doctor about possible treatments for acid reflux;
- avoid lying down or reclining for 2 to 3 hours after eating;
- try to eat your last meal 3 hours before going to bed;
- exercise in the morning before you eat;
- drink liquids between meals, not with them; and
- make sure that constipation is resolved.

FOUR WEEKS TO CALM ACID REFLUX

Please note in the meal plans that follow, you should plan to eat twice for every meal, 2 to 3 hours apart—so eat breakfast at 6 a.m. and 8 a.m., for example. You don't need to make two recipes for every meal, just split one serving into two sittings.

WEEK ONE

Be sure to use the Plan A modifications for all recipes listed here.

MONDAY

Breakfast: 2 slices toast, using Udi's gluten-free sandwich bread, each slice topped with 1 teaspoon peanut butter

Lunch: Potato Leek Soup, page 84

Dinner: Savory Vegetable Soup, page 79

TUESDAY

Breakfast: Maple-Cinnamon Oatmeal, page 66

Lunch: Turkey sandwich on Udi's gluten-free sandwich bread with 1 teaspoon Dijon mustard

Dinner: Veggie-Stuffed Trout, page 122

WEDNESDAY

Breakfast: Blueberry Muffins, page 106

Lunch: Kale Salad with Feta Cheese and Walnuts, page 88

Dinner: Pork Chops with Rhubarb Sauce, page 143

THURSDAY

Breakfast: 2 slices toast, using Udi's gluten-free sandwich bread, each slice topped with 1 teaspoon peanut butter

Lunch: Tuna salad sandwich made with 2 teaspoons Mayonnaise, page 178, and 2 teaspoons plain yogurt mixed with 3 ounces water-packed tuna, drained, and served on Udi's gluten-free sandwich bread.

Dinner: Orange Chicken and Veggie Stir-Fry, page 140, and steamed rice

FRIDAY

Breakfast: Zucchini, Red Pepper, and Egg Scramble, page 73

Lunch: Turkey-ham sandwich on Udi's gluten-free sandwich bread with 2 teaspoons Dijon mustard

Dinner: Pork Tenderloin with Asian Slaw, page 142

SATURDAY

Breakfast: Potato Hash with Fried Egg, page 72

Lunch: Shrimp Fried Rice, page 116

Dinner: Bistro Burgers, page 150

SUNDAY

Breakfast: Blueberry Pancakes, page 67

Lunch: Ground Turkey Stir-Fry, page 137

Dinner: Cinnamon Shrimp, page 132

SNACKS FOR THE WEEK

Baked Green Bean "Fries," page 102

Yogurt with Flaxseed and Blueberries, page 104

Sweet and Spicy Pecans, page 98

WEEK TWO

Be sure to use the Plan A modifications for all recipes listed here.

MONDAY

Breakfast: 2 slices toast, using Udi's gluten-free sandwich bread, each slice topped with 1 teaspoon peanut butter

Lunch: Egg salad sandwich: Chop 1 hardboiled egg and 2 hardboiled egg whites; mix with ½ grated carrot, 2 teaspoons Mayonnaise, page 178, 2 teaspoons plain low-fat lactose-free yogurt, and 1 teaspoon Dijon mustard; and serve on Udi's gluten-free sandwich bread.

Dinner: Shrimp Scampi with Zucchini Noodles, page 117

TUESDAY

Breakfast: Lemon Dutch Baby, page 68

Lunch: Ground Beef and Veggie Soup, page 86

Dinner: Turkey Piccata, page 136, with steamed rice and veggies

WEDNESDAY

Breakfast: Scrambled eggs made from 3 egg whites and 1 egg yolk

Lunch: Purchased rotisserie chicken with Potato Salad, page 93

Dinner: Maple-Soy Glazed Salmon with Tri-Pepper Sauté, page 126

THURSDAY

Breakfast: Bacon and Potato Frittata, page 70

Lunch: Baked potato with 2 teaspoons butter, 1 tablespoon grated Cheddar cheese, and shredded rotisserie chicken

Dinner: Clam Chowder (double batch), page 80

FRIDAY

Breakfast: Maple-Cinnamon Oatmeal, page 66

Lunch: Chopped Salad with Basil Vinaigrette, page 90

Dinner: Purchased rotisserie chicken with Warm Spinach Salad, page 89

SATURDAY

Breakfast: Ham Strata, page 75

Lunch: Leftover Clam Chowder

Dinner: Halibut with Rice and Pineapple Salsa, page 130

SUNDAY

Breakfast: Spiced Orange French Toast, page 69

Lunch: Broiled fish and Cucumber Salad with Asian Ginger Vinaigrette, page 91

Dinner: Hearty Meatloaf, page 144, with Loaded Smashed Potatoes, page 110

SNACKS FOR THE WEEK

Deviled Eggs, page 97

Baked Zucchini Chips, page 105

Spiced Roasted Pepitas, page 96

Blueberry Muffins, page 106

Baked Green Bean "Fries," page 102

WEEK THREE

Be sure to use the Plan A modifications for all recipes listed here.

MONDAY

Breakfast: 2 slices toast, using Udi's gluten-free sandwich bread, spread with ¼ avocado

Lunch: Sandwich made with Udi's gluten-free sandwich bread, 1 tablespoon peanut butter (or Sunflower Butter, page 187), and half a banana

Dinner: Savory Vegetable Soup, page 79

TUESDAY

Breakfast: Blueberry Pancakes, page 67

Lunch: Chicken Soup with Zucchini Noodles, page 82

Dinner: Fish and Chips, page 129

WEDNESDAY

Breakfast: Blueberry Muffins, page 106

Lunch: 2 slices Udi's gluten-free sandwich bread spread with Zucchini Hummus (¼ cup per day max), page 101, and topped with sliced cucumbers

Dinner: Shrimp and Grits, page 114

THURSDAY

Breakfast: Egg white scramble (use 3 whites) and ½ slice toast made from Udi's gluten-free sandwich bread spread with 1 teaspoon butter

Lunch: Simple Crab Salad, page 120

Dinner: Arroz con Pollo, page 141

FRIDAY

Breakfast: Spiced Orange French Toast, page 69

Lunch: Chef's salad made with iceberg lettuce, chopped turkey, and 1 carrot, dressed with 2 tablespoons Basil Vinaigrette, page 185

Dinner: Bistro Burgers, page 150

SATURDAY

Breakfast: Bacon and Potato Frittata, page 70

Lunch: Savory Vegetable Soup, page 79

Dinner: Cottage Pie, page 154

SUNDAY

Breakfast: Lemon Dutch Baby, page 68

Lunch: Baked Mediterranean Turkey Meatballs *without* the Roasted Red Pepper Sauce, page 151; make a dipping sauce from plain coconut yogurt and grated cucumber instead.

Dinner: Pan-Seared Scallops with Orange Aioli, page 124

SNACKS FOR THE WEEK

Maple Corn Bread, page 111

Baked Potato Chips, page 99

Zucchini Hummus (¼ cup per day max), page 101

Hardboiled egg whites

Spiced Roasted Pepitas, page 96

WEEK FOUR

Be sure to use the Plan A modifications for all recipes listed here.

MONDAY

Breakfast: Maple-Cinnamon Oatmeal, page 66

Lunch: Ground Beef and Veggie Soup, page 86

Dinner: Turkey Meatballs with Gingered Bok Choy, page 138

TUESDAY

Breakfast: Ginger Melon Smoothie, page 64

Lunch: Broiled chicken breast and Roasted Vegetable Salad, page 92

Dinner: Veggie-Stuffed Trout, page 122

WEDNESDAY

Breakfast: Blueberry Muffins, page 106

Lunch: Roast beef sandwich on Udi's gluten-free sandwich bread with 1½ teaspoons Mayonnaise, page 178, and 1 teaspoon Dijon mustard

Dinner: Cinnamon Shrimp, page 132

THURSDAY

Breakfast: Zucchini, Red Pepper, and Egg Scramble, page 73

Lunch: Savory Vegetable Soup, page 79, and Maple Corn Bread, page 111

Dinner: Lemon Pepper Cod, *without* the pepper, with Roasted Root Veggies, page 118

FRIDAY

Breakfast: Leftover Blueberry Muffins

Lunch: 2 hardboiled egg whites and carrot sticks

Dinner: Orange Chicken and Veggie Stir-Fry, page 140

SATURDAY

Breakfast: Potato Hash with Fried Egg, page 72

Lunch: Hearty Fish Stew, page 128

Dinner: Maple-Soy Glazed Salmon, *without* the Tri-Pepper Sauté, page 126, and Ambrosia Salad, page 87

SUNDAY

Breakfast: Lemon Dutch Baby, page 68

Lunch: Bistro Burgers, page 150

Dinner: Steamer Clams with Fennel in Broth, page 121

SNACKS FOR THE WEEK

Spiced Roasted Pepitas, page 96

Blueberry Muffins, page 106

Sesame Kale Chips, page 100

Sweet and Spicy Pecans, page 98

Yogurt with Flaxseed and Blueberries, page 104

The
LOW-FODMAP
MEAL PLAN FOR IBS-C

If your primary form of IBS is IBS-C (with constipation), then you may need to make some minor modifications to your diet. For the most part, the recipes for the IBS-C diet can be used as written unless modifications are specified. However, you may need to make some of the following modifications to manage your particular symptoms.

Recipes that are appropriate for managing IBS-C (or can be modified to be appropriate by following the "for Plan C" recipe tip) will be designated with a "C" icon.

ADD FIBER

If you suffer from constipation, fiber is your friend because it provides bulk to the foods you eat, which helps alleviate constipation. Therefore, choose higher fiber versions of the foods. For example:

- Leave vegetable and fruit peels on whenever possible, because they are an excellent source of fiber.

- Choose higher fiber grains, such as brown rice or quinoa, in place of white rice.

- Incorporate nuts and seeds into meals, such as chia seeds and flaxseed.

INCREASE FIBER INTAKE GRADUALLY

You don't want to shock your body with too much fiber all of a sudden. If you've been consuming a low-fiber diet up till now, increase your fiber intake gradually. Consuming too much fiber too quickly can induce gas and bloating—symptoms you're trying to get rid of.

DRINK PLENTY OF FLUIDS

Fluid consumption can also help alleviate constipation. Try to drink about eight cups of water per day and avoid caffeine, which can act as a diuretic and flush the fluids out of your system when consumed in large amounts.

CHALLENGES

Most challenges with this version of the low-FODMAP diet come from pain and cramping associated with constipation, as well as gas and bloating from increasing fiber content too quickly. Increase your fiber gradually over a few weeks. If you do this too quickly, you may notice stomach upset that turns to diarrhea. It may also, then, be a challenge to take in enough fluid, so carry water with you and sip it throughout the day.

TWO WEEKS TO RELIEVE IBS-C

Follow the IBS-C plan for 2 weeks before changing to the regular IBS plan for 2 weeks more. If you develop diarrhea, switch to the IBS-D plan until you have reached balance.

WEEK ONE

Be sure to use the Plan C recipe adaptations for recipes listed here.

MONDAY

Breakfast: Dark Chocolate and Banana Smoothie, page 60

Lunch: Potato Leek Soup, page 84

Dinner: Spaghetti and Meatballs, page 146, and a green salad made with romaine lettuce and tomatoes and dressed with Basil Vinaigrette, page 185

TUESDAY

Breakfast: Maple-Cinnamon Oatmeal, page 66

Lunch: Turkey sandwich on Udi's whole-grain gluten-free sandwich bread with 1 teaspoon Dijon mustard

Dinner: Veggie-Stuffed Trout, page 122, and steamed brown rice

WEDNESDAY

Breakfast: PB&J Smoothie, page 62

Lunch: Kale Salad with Feta Cheese and Walnuts, page 88

Dinner: Pork Chops with Rhubarb Sauce, page 143, and steamed quinoa

THURSDAY

Breakfast: Spiced Orange French Toast, page 69

Lunch: Tuna salad sandwich made with 1 tablespoon Mayonnaise, page 178, and 3 ounces water-packed tuna, drained, topped with baby spinach, and served on Udi's whole-grain gluten-free bread.

Dinner: Orange Chicken and Veggie Stir-Fry, page 140, and steamed brown rice

FRIDAY

Breakfast: Zucchini, Red Pepper, and Egg Scramble, page 73

Lunch: Easy Tomato Soup, page 78, with ½ cup cooked quinoa stirred in

Dinner: Pork Tenderloin with Asian Slaw, page 142, and steamed brown rice

SATURDAY

Breakfast: Potato Hash with Fried Egg, page 72 (leave the skin on the potatoes)

Lunch: Shrimp Fried Rice, page 116, made with brown rice

Dinner: Zucchini Lasagna, page 152, and Warm Spinach Salad, page 89

SUNDAY

Breakfast: Blueberry Pancakes, page 67

Lunch: Ground Turkey Stir-Fry, page 137, with steamed brown rice

Dinner: Fish Curry, page 133, with steamed brown rice or quinoa

SNACKS FOR THE WEEK

Zucchini Hummus (¼ cup per day max), page 101, with veggies

Yogurt with Flaxseed and Blueberries, page 104

WEEK TWO

Be sure to use the Plan C recipe adaptations for recipes listed here.

MONDAY

Breakfast: Orange Chia Smoothie, page 63, with 2 extra tablespoons chia seeds

Lunch: Egg salad sandwich: chop 2 hardboiled eggs and mix with ½ grated carrot, 1 tablespoon Mayonnaise, page 178, 1 teaspoon Dijon mustard, and serve on Udi's whole-grain gluten-free sandwich bread

Dinner: Shrimp Scampi with Zucchini Noodles, page 117, and a salad made with kale and dressed with Basil Vinaigrette, page 185

TUESDAY

Breakfast: PB&J Smoothie, page 62

Lunch: Ground Beef and Veggie Soup, page 86, with ½ cup cooked quinoa stirred in

Dinner: Turkey Piccata, page 136, with rice and veggies, using brown rice

WEDNESDAY

Breakfast: Dark Chocolate and Banana Smoothie, page 60

Lunch: Purchased rotisserie chicken on Kale Salad with Feta Cheese and Walnuts, page 88

Dinner: Maple-Soy Glazed Salmon with Tri-Pepper Sauté, page 126, and steamed brown rice

THURSDAY

Breakfast: Bacon and Potato Frittata, page 70

Lunch: Skin-on baked potato topped with 1 tablespoon butter (or butter substitute), 1 ounce grated cheese, and shredded rotisserie chicken.

Dinner: Minestrone, page 83, with ½ cup steamed brown rice stirred in

FRIDAY

Breakfast: Maple-Cinnamon Oatmeal, page 66

Lunch: Chopped Salad with Basil Vinaigrette, page 90

Dinner: Purchased rotisserie chicken with Warm Spinach Salad, page 89

SATURDAY

Breakfast: Ham Strata, page 75, and 1 slice toast using Udi's whole-grain gluten-free sandwich bread

Lunch: Broiled chicken breast and Roasted Vegetable Salad, page 92

Dinner: Halibut with Rice and Pineapple Salsa, page 130

SUNDAY

Breakfast: Spiced Orange French Toast, page 69

Lunch: Broiled fish with Cucumber Salad with Asian Ginger Vinaigrette, page 91

Dinner: Hearty Meatloaf, page 144, with Loaded Smashed Potatoes, page 110

SNACKS FOR THE WEEK

Maple Corn Bread, page 111

Baked Zucchini Chips, page 105

Spiced Roasted Pepitas, page 96

Chips and Salsa, page 109

Blueberry Muffins, page 106

The
LOW-FODMAP
MEAL PLAN FOR IBD OR IBS-D

For people with IBS-D (diarrhea dominant) or IBD in remission, it's especially important to be gentle on your stomach. Most recipes in this book can be adapted for IBS-D and IBD in remission, and it's important you listen to your body to determine the changes it needs. Some specific tips for sufferers of IBD and IBS-D follow. Recipes that are appropriate for IBS-D or IBD in remission (or that can be modified to be appropriate by following the "For Plan D" recipe tip) will be designated with a "D" icon.

AVOID SKIPPING MEALS

Eat small meals or snacks every 3 to 4 hours, even if you aren't feeling well. This is important to replace lost nutrients and fluids.

DRINK PLENTY OF FLUIDS

Water is your best bet here. It is gentle on your stomach and it will rehydrate you from fluids lost during diarrhea. Aim for at least eight cups of water daily, sipped throughout the day.

DECREASE FIBER INTAKE

High fiber increases frequency of bowel movements, which is the opposite of what you want when you have diarrhea.

Therefore, it's important to minimize fiber intake while diarrhea is present by

- peeling fruits and vegetables;
- using "white" versions of grains such as light-colored flours, white gluten-free bread, and white rice; and
- as you add fiber, add only one fiber food at a time to see how your body tolerates it. For instance, try ¼ cup cooked brown rice and notice how your body tolerates it. If you return to loose stools, go back to low-fiber foods and try again another time.

LIMIT SUGAR, SUGAR SUBSTITUTES, AND CAFFEINE

Both sugar and caffeine can stimulate the bowels, which can be an issue if you're suffering from diarrhea. Therefore, avoid the following:

- Alcoholic beverages
- Artificial sweeteners and sugar alcohols
- Caffeinated tea
- Chocolate
- Coffee
- Energy drinks
- Fruit juices
- Soda and diet soda

LIMIT DAIRY AND FAT

The lactose in dairy products may contribute to bloating, gas, and diarrhea. While the recipes in this book limit dairy, you may need to avoid it completely until you have your symptoms under control.

MODIFY TEXTURES

You may also wish to modify the textures of your food. You can do this by

- choosing soft fruits or cooked fruits;
- cooking proteins in liquid to make them very soft;
- cooking vegetables very well;
- puréeing foods, as needed; and
- using nut and seed butters instead of whole nuts and seeds.

POSSIBLE CHALLENGES

Here are some possible challenges and tips to help you manage when diarrhea is your predominate symptom.

YOU DON'T FEEL LIKE EATING

If this is the case, eat small meals regularly, and modify the textures of the meals you eat so the foods are soft and soothing.

SPICY OR FLAVORFUL FOOD IRRITATES YOUR STOMACH

If this describes you, limit spices in your foods, sticking to mild or slightly sweet spices such as cinnamon, ginger, or herbs.

YOU FEEL NAUSEATED

Again, alter the texture of foods to make them very soft, and eat small amounts. This can help. Ginger and fennel are especially good for upset stomachs, so incorporate these flavors into your foods.

TWO WEEKS TO RELIEVE IBD/IBS-D

If you're struggling with IBS-D, diarrhea, or nausea associated with IBS or IBD, then try this meal plan. As symptoms abate, switch to the basic IBS meal plan (see page 37), returning to this one as needed.

WEEK ONE

Be sure you use thePlan D adaptations for the recipes listed.

MONDAY

Breakfast: PB&J Smoothie, page 62

Lunch: Potato Leek Soup, page 84

Dinner: Cottage Pie, page 154

TUESDAY

Breakfast: Maple-Cinnamon Oatmeal, page 66

Lunch: Baked potato (don't eat the skin) with 2 tablespoons fat-free, lactose-free yogurt and steamed chicken breast

Dinner: Veggie-Stuffed Trout, page 122, and steamed white rice

WEDNESDAY

Breakfast: Ginger Melon Smoothie, page 64

Lunch: Easy Tomato Soup, page 78

Dinner: Simple Crab Salad, page 120

THURSDAY

Breakfast: Spiced Orange French Toast, page 69

Lunch: Tuna salad made with 4 ounces water-packed tuna, drained, 2 tablespoons Mayonnaise, page 178, 1 teaspoon Dijon mustard, and sea salt

Dinner: Maple-Soy Glazed Salmon with Tri-Pepper Sauté, page 126, and steamed white rice

FRIDAY

Breakfast: Zucchini, Red Pepper, and Egg Scramble, page 73

Lunch: Chicken salad made from 3 ounces steamed chicken breast, 2 tablespoons Mayonnaise, page 178, steamed carrots, 1 teaspoon dried tarragon, and sea salt.

Dinner: Pork Tenderloin with Asian Slaw, page 142, and steamed white rice

SATURDAY

Breakfast: Potato Hash with Fried Egg, page 72

Lunch: Shrimp Fried Rice, page 116

Dinner: Purchased rotisserie chicken and Loaded Smashed Potatoes, page 110

SUNDAY

Breakfast: Blueberry Pancakes, page 67

Lunch: Ground Turkey Stir-Fry, page 137, with steamed white rice

Dinner: Fish Curry, page 133

SNACKS FOR THE WEEK

Ambrosia Salad, page 87

Zucchini Hummus (¼ cup daily), page 101

Yogurt with Flaxseed and Blueberries, *without* the flaxseed, page 104

WEEK TWO

Be sure you use the Plan D adaptations for the recipes listed.

MONDAY

Breakfast: Orange Chia Smoothie, page 63

Lunch: Egg salad sandwich: chop
2 hardboiled eggs and mix with
1 tablespoon Mayonnaise, page 178,
1 teaspoon Dijon mustard, and serve on
Udi's gluten-free sandwich bread

Dinner: Shrimp and Grits, page 114

TUESDAY

Breakfast: Piña Colada Smoothie, page 61

Lunch: Ground Beef and Veggie Soup,
page 86

Dinner: Turkey Piccata, page 136, with
steamed white rice and veggies

WEDNESDAY

Breakfast: Ginger-Melon Smoothie,
page 64

Lunch: Purchased rotisserie chicken
and steamed white rice

Dinner: Pan-Seared Scallops with
Orange Aioli, page 124

THURSDAY

Breakfast: Bacon and Potato
Frittata, page 70

Lunch: Baked potato (don't eat the skin)
with 1 tablespoon butter, 1 ounce
fat-free grated cheese, and shredded
rotisserie chicken

Dinner: Minestrone, page 83

FRIDAY

Breakfast: Maple-Cinnamon
Oatmeal, page 66

Lunch: Simple Crab Salad, page 120

Dinner: Clam Chowder, page 80

SATURDAY

Breakfast: Ham Strata, page 75

Lunch: Broiled chicken breast with
Roasted Vegetable Salad, page 92

Dinner: Halibut with Rice and
Pineapple Salsa, page 130

SUNDAY

Breakfast: Spiced Orange French
Toast, page 69

Lunch: Broiled fish with steamed carrots
and steamed white rice

Dinner: Hearty Meatloaf, page 144, with
Loaded Smashed Potatoes, page 110

SNACKS FOR THE WEEK

Maple Corn Bread, page 111

Baked Zucchini Chips, page 105

Blueberry Muffins, page 106

PRACTICING SELF-COMPASSION

Undertaking a new way of eating isn't easy, so treat yourself with kindness and compassion. Things won't always go perfectly, so forgive and encourage yourself as you make this journey to better health.

HEED YOUR BODY'S SIGNALS

If you've been sick and symptomatic for a long time, chances are you've tuned out the signals your body sends you to some extent just to make it through every day. But it's necessary to understand that your body sends signals for a reason: It's trying to communicate with you. Throughout this process, it's important to learn to listen to your body and do what it asks. Offer gentle exercise, but don't force heavy exercise if you don't feel up to it. Drink when you're thirsty, eat when you're hungry, and rest when your body tells you it needs to take a moment to recharge.

GET PLENTY OF SLEEP

We live in a world where sleeping is often viewed as a weakness—but it is extremely necessary for healing a body. Dealing with chronic illness can be debilitating and exhausting, and as your body heals, it will need sleep to restore itself. So allow plenty of time to sleep. Go to bed earlier in the evening, if necessary. Create a healthy sleep environment free of ambient light and light emitted from electronics, noise, and at a comfortable temperature. Use your bed only for sleep, and go to bed and get up at the same time daily. Establish a sleep routine. These good sleep habits will help you get the sleep you need as your body recovers.

GIVE YOURSELF A BREAK

Change can be difficult, so you need to be kind to yourself. You may experience some resistance to changes in your diet. At times, you may decide this diet isn't for you and succumb to a craving. When these thoughts, feelings, and actions occur, be forgiving. Slipping isn't failing, and you can get back to your low-FODMAP diet. Be kind in how you talk to yourself. If you slip, talk to yourself like you would to a friend or loved one. Every moment of every day provides the opportunity to choose anew.

ENGAGE IN GENTLE AND SELF-LOVING LEISURE PURSUITS

Nobody wants to work, work, work all the time. Give yourself time to experience the joy in life: get out and do things you love. Go on a walk. Engage in meditation. Do a craft. Enjoy a bath. Write a poem. Take a yoga class. Read a book. Do things that help you focus on the moment.

REST WHEN YOU DON'T FEEL WELL

If you don't feel well, rest. Take the time to allow your body to heal. There's no "right" way to do this—only the way that is most supportive of your needs and symptoms.

ENJOY SUPPORT

Build a group of supportive friends and family around you. Spend time with your tribe, laughing and enjoying life. Or, join a local group or class that shares your interests. While many social rituals revolve around food, it doesn't need to be stressful for you. Bring your own foods and beverages with you to such gatherings and enjoy the fellowship that comes from engaging with friends.

A TIME TO HEAL

Remember, the diet as written here is temporary, intended to treat your body gently as you heal and then allow you to find a way to eat that works for your unique health needs. You should begin to notice relief of your symptoms within the first week or two. Keep track of this so you can remind yourself how far you've come. By choosing to follow a low-FODMAP diet, you've taken the first step toward finding your way to eat so you can lead a vibrant, healthy, symptom-free life.

The LOW-FODMAP RECIPES

2

All recipes in the following chapters are designed for a low-FODMAP diet and appropriate for the "basic" low-FODMAP meal plan—whether by nature of the ingredients used or the serving size. Recipe labels can help you determine whether these recipes are also appropriate for other coexisting conditions, as well as for the type of IBS you experience.

A **PLAN A** recipes are good for those experiencing symptoms of gastroesophageal reflux disease and acid reflux in addition to their IBS symptoms.

B **PLAN B** recipes are for those experiencing general IBS symptoms.

C **PLAN C** recipes are best for people whose IBS presents predominately with constipation.

D **PLAN D** recipes are best for people whose IBS presents predominately with diarrhea or for those who also have IBD.

MAKE AHEAD recipes can be prepped or completely made ahead of time

ONE-POT meals can be made in a single pot or bowl.

PORTABLE recipes are easy to transport for meals on the go.

VEGETARIAN OR VEGAN recipes contain no meat or no animal products.

You'll also find tips for making recipes appropriate for one or more of the listed categories, as well as making them free of what are called the **BIG 8 ALLERGENS** (milk, eggs, fish, shellfish, tree nuts, peanuts, wheat, and soybeans), when possible.

To make sure you do not go over the allowed amount of FODMAPs, pay attention to the number of servings each recipe makes, and eat only one serving. For example, if a recipe serves four people, eat only one-fourth of what that recipe makes.

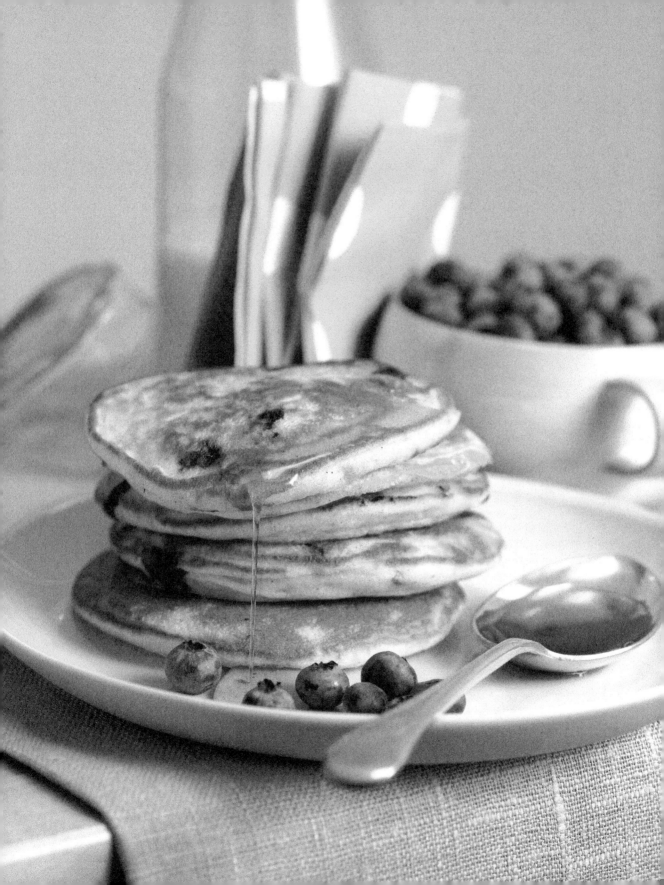

3

SMOOTHIES AND BREAKFAST

DARK CHOCOLATE AND BANANA SMOOTHIE

MAKE AHEAD | **ONE-POT** | **PORTABLE** | **VEGAN** Smoothies are a great way to start your day. Loaded with nutrition, they are quick and easy to make, portable, and delicious. This smoothie is an excellent source of potassium, and the addition of flaxseed adds omega-3 fatty acids that can help reduce inflammation. This recipe makes two servings, so you can share with someone else or refrigerate leftovers overnight and have your second serving for breakfast tomorrow or a snack later. *Serves 2*

PREP 5 minutes
COOK 0 minutes

2 cups unsweetened rice milk

1 banana, peeled

2 tablespoons unsweetened dark cocoa powder

2 tablespoons flaxseed

1 tablespoon pure maple syrup

1 packet stevia (optional)

¼ cup crushed ice

In a blender, combine the rice milk, banana, cocoa, flaxseed, maple syrup, stevia (if using), and ice. Process until smooth and serve.

for **PLAN A** This smoothie is not GERD-friendly. Eliminate the cocoa powder and add 1 teaspoon alcohol-free vanilla extract for a banana smoothie instead.

for **PLAN D** Eliminate the flaxseed to reduce the fiber content of this smoothie.

PER SERVING Calories: 248; Total fat: 5g; Saturated fat: <1g; Carbohydrates: 50g; Fiber: 5g; Protein: 3g

PIÑA COLADA SMOOTHIE

MAKE AHEAD | **ONE-POT** | **PORTABLE** | **VEGAN** A tasty tropical smoothie helps energize your body and your taste buds in the morning. If you're feeling adventurous, add a dollop (about ¼ teaspoon) of rum extract. Although it isn't necessary, it punches up the flavor and makes you feel like you're starting your day poolside with an umbrella drink in your hand. *Serves 2*

PREP 5 minutes
COOK 0 minutes

2 cups canned full-fat coconut milk

1 cup canned crushed pineapple, drained

¼ teaspoon rum extract (optional)

1 packet stevia (optional)

½ cup crushed ice

In a blender, combine the coconut milk, pineapple, rum extract (if using), stevia (if using), and ice. Process until smooth and serve.

for **PLAN A** Pineapple may be a GERD trigger, so avoid this recipe.

for **PLAN C** If you struggle with constipation, add 2 tablespoons chia seeds to increase the fiber content.

PER SERVING Calories: 176; Total fat: 12g; Saturated fat: 11g; Carbohydrates: 20g; Fiber: 1g; Protein: 3g

PB&J SMOOTHIE

MAKE AHEAD | **ONE-POT** | **PORTABLE** | **VEGAN** Who doesn't love peanut butter and jelly? This simple smoothie will take you right back to your favorite childhood sandwich, but one full of nutritious ingredients such as fresh berries and creamy nut butter. One sip and you'll feel like a kid again. *Serves 2*

PREP 5 minutes
COOK 0 minutes

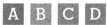

2 cups unsweetened rice milk

¼ cup fresh blueberries

2 tablespoons peanut butter

1 packet stevia (optional)

½ cup crushed ice

In a blender, combine the rice milk, blueberries, peanut butter, stevia (if using), and ice. Process until smooth and serve.

for **PLAN A** Reduce the peanut butter to 1 tablespoon; reduce the serving size by half or eat 1 full serving in 2 meals, 2 to 3 hours apart, to avoid overfilling your stomach.

for **PLAN C** If you struggle with constipation, add 2 tablespoons flaxseed to increase the fiber content.

SUBSTITUTION TIP If you're allergic to peanuts, replace the peanut butter with Sunflower Butter (page 187).

PER SERVING Calories: 233; Total fat: 10g; Saturated fat: 2g; Carbohydrates: 34g; Fiber: 2g; Protein: 5g

ORANGE CHIA SMOOTHIE

MAKE AHEAD | ONE-POT | PORTABLE | VEGAN Remember those creamy, dreamy, orangey frozen treats on a stick when you were a kid? Those orange–vanilla ice cream treats were delicious and refreshing, showing you just how tasty the flavor combination could be. This smoothie makes a nutritious and satisfying breakfast and will remind you of the delicious flavors of those ice creams. *Serves 2*

PREP 5 minutes
COOK 0 minutes

1½ cups unsweetened rice milk

Juice of 2 oranges

½ cup unsweetened plain coconut yogurt

2 tablespoons chia seeds

½ teaspoon vanilla extract

1 packet stevia (optional)

½ cup crushed ice

In a blender, combine the rice milk, orange juice, yogurt, chia seeds, vanilla, stevia (if using), and ice. Process until smooth and serve.

for **PLAN A** The acid in orange juice can trigger GERD, so substitute either ½ teaspoon orange extract or the zest of half an orange to get the orange flavor without the acid. If you leave out the orange juice, increase the rice milk to 2 cups. Reduce the serving size by half or eat 1 full serving in 2 meals, 2 to 3 hours apart, to avoid overfilling your stomach.

for **PLAN D** Eliminate the chia seeds.

PER SERVING Calories: 235; Total fat: 7g; Saturated fat: 1g; Carbohydrates: 37g; Fiber: 6g; Protein: 6g

GINGER MELON SMOOTHIE

MAKE AHEAD | **ONE-POT** | **PORTABLE** | **VEGAN** Ginger and melon are especially soothing for people with GERD and acid reflux, so this smoothie is a good one to have if you notice acid flare-ups. Both ingredients settle and cool the stomach, which makes them helpful for all kinds of bowel conditions. Ginger also adds lots of flavor. To prep the ginger, use a rasp-style grater. *Serves 2*

PREP 5 minutes
COOK 0 minutes

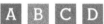

2 cups unsweetened rice milk

1 cup cubed cantaloupe

1 cup cubed
honeydew melon

1 teaspoon grated peeled
fresh ginger

Pinch ground nutmeg

1 packet stevia (optional)

½ cup crushed ice

In a blender, combine the rice milk, cantaloupe, honeydew, ginger, nutmeg, stevia (if using), and ice. Process until smooth and serve.

for **PLAN A** Reduce the serving size by half or eat 1 full serving in 2 meals, 2 to 3 hours apart, to avoid overfilling your stomach.

for **PLAN C** Add 2 tablespoons flaxseed for additional fiber.

PER SERVING Calories: 181; Total fat: 2g; Saturated fat: 0g; Carbohydrates: 39g; Fiber: 2g; Protein: 2g

SIMPLE GREENS SMOOTHIE

MAKE AHEAD | **ONE-POT** | **PORTABLE** | **VEGAN** Green smoothies are an excellent source of fiber, and adding a little fruit provides sweetness. While the recipe calls for raw greens, you can also steam them or use frozen spinach so the smoothie blends easier in a lower powered blender. *Serves 2*

PREP 5 minutes
COOK 0 minutes

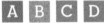

1 cup fresh spinach, washed

1 cup kale, washed

1½ cups unsweetened rice milk

½ cup freshly squeezed orange juice

½ banana

Pinch ground cinnamon

4 ice cubes

½ cup crushed ice

In a blender, combine the spinach, kale, rice milk, orange juice, banana, cinnamon, and ice. Blend until smooth and serve.

for **PLAN A** Eliminate the orange juice and replace it with ½ cup unsweetened rice milk. Replace the cinnamon with ground ginger and add a packet of stevia for a bit of sweetness.

for **PLAN D** Steam the vegetables (and then cool completely) before adding them to the smoothie. Beware that this smoothie may have a bit too much roughage for someone with IBD.

PER SERVING Calories: 160; Total fat: 2g; Saturated fat: 0g; Carbohydrates: 33g; Fiber: 2g; Protein: 2g

MAPLE-CINNAMON OATMEAL

ONE-POT | **VEGAN** There's just something so satisfying and stick-to-your ribs about oatmeal for breakfast. When working with oats, it's important to purchase oats that are certified gluten-free, because oats are often processed in places that also process wheat and other grains. *Serves 4*

PREP 5 minutes
COOK 25 minutes

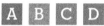

3½ cups boiling water

1 cup steel cut oats

½ cup unsweetened rice milk

2 tablespoons pure maple syrup

1 tablespoon packed brown sugar

1 teaspoon ground cinnamon

Zest of ½ orange

Pinch sea salt

1. In a medium saucepan over high heat, mix the water, oats, rice milk, maple syrup, sugar, cinnamon, orange zest, and sea salt.

2. Bring to a boil and then reduce the heat to medium-low. Simmer for about 25 minutes, stirring occasionally, until the oats are soft.

for **PLAN A** Replace the cinnamon with ½ teaspoon ground ginger and ¼ teaspoon ground nutmeg. Reduce the serving size by half or eat 1 full serving in 2 meals, 2 to 3 hours apart, to avoid overfilling your stomach.

for **PLAN D** and **BIG 8 ALLERGENS** Replace the oats with yellow cornmeal and use 1½ cups cornmeal to 3 cups water. Simmer, stirring, for about 7 minutes. All other ingredients remain the same.

PER SERVING Calories: 210; Total fat: 3g; Saturated fat: 0g; Carbohydrates: 41g; Fiber: 5g; Protein: 7g

BLUEBERRY PANCAKES

PORTABLE | VEGETARIAN Pancakes are one of the easiest foods to make using gluten-free flour because you want a tender crumb, and so the sticky, binding power of gluten isn't needed. These blueberry pancakes are light, fluffy, and delicious—with or without syrup. If you use maple syrup, select pure maple syrup and limit it to 1 tablespoon. *Serves 4*

PREP 10 minutes
COOK 10 minutes

2⅓ cups King Arthur gluten-free flour

2 teaspoons gluten-free baking powder

1 packet stevia (optional)

½ teaspoon sea salt

2 large eggs

½ very ripe banana, mashed

4 tablespoons canola oil, plus more for the pan

2 cups unsweetened rice milk

1 cup fresh blueberries

1. In a large bowl, mix the flour, baking powder, stevia (if using), and sea salt.

2. In a medium bowl, whisk the eggs, banana, canola oil, and rice milk. Add the egg mixture to the flour mixture, stirring until just combined.

3. Gently fold in the blueberries.

4. Heat a nonstick skillet over medium-high heat. Coat the hot pan with canola oil.

5. Working in batches, pour the batter into the hot pan, 2 tablespoons at a time. Cook for about 3 minutes until the pancakes bubble. Flip and cook for about 2 minutes more until browned.

for **PLAN A** Reduce the canola oil to 2 tablespoons and add 1 more egg. Reduce the serving size by half or eat 1 full serving in 2 meals, 2 to 3 hours apart, to avoid overfilling your stomach.

for **PLAN C** Add 2 tablespoons ground flaxseed for additional fiber.

BIG 8 ALLERGENS Replace the eggs with flaxseed eggs (see page 28).

PER SERVING Calories: 514; Total fat: 18g; Saturated fat: 13g; Carbohydrates: 78g; Fiber: 3g; Protein: 11g

LEMON DUTCH BABY

VEGETARIAN A Dutch baby is a magical pancake that turns golden and puffed when you cook it. This one is made with lemon zest so it's packed with bright lemon flavor. You can also sprinkle it with lemon juice and powdered sugar after it is cooked for even more citrus flavor. *Serves 4*

PREP 5 minutes
COOK 15 minutes

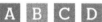

2 tablespoons canola oil

8 large eggs

1 cup unsweetened rice milk

¼ cup arrowroot powder

¼ cup coconut flour

1 teaspoon vanilla extract

Pinch ground nutmeg

Pinch sea salt

Zest of 1 lemon

1. Preheat the oven to 425°F.

2. Put the canola oil into a 9-by-13-inch baking dish and put the dish in the oven while you work.

3. In a blender, process the eggs for about 1 minute on high until they are combined.

4. Add the rice milk, arrowroot powder, coconut flour, vanilla, nutmeg, sea salt, and lemon zest. Blend for about 30 seconds on high until well mixed. Carefully pour the batter into the prepared pan.

5. Bake for about 15 minutes until puffy and set.

for **PLAN A** Reduce the oil to 1 tablespoon. Reduce the serving size by half or eat 1 full serving in 2 meals, 2 to 3 hours apart, to avoid overfilling your stomach.

for **PLAN C** Top with fresh berries to increase the fiber content.

BIG 8 ALLERGENS If you're allergic to eggs, there's not really a substitute here, so avoid this recipe.

PER SERVING Calories: 240; Total fat: 18g; Saturated fat: 10g; Carbohydrates: 9g; Fiber: <1g; Protein: 12g

SPICED ORANGE FRENCH TOAST

PORTABLE | VEGETARIAN French toast is a family favorite—and for good reason. With custardy bread and delicious spices, French toast is delicious by itself or with a little pure maple syrup (don't use more than 1 tablespoon). You can even take French toast (minus the syrup) with you as a meal-on-the-go option. *Serves 4*

PREP 5 minutes
COOK 15 minutes

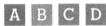

6 large eggs

2 cups unsweetened rice milk

Zest of 1 orange

1 packet stevia

½ teaspoon ground cinnamon

⅛ teaspoon ground nutmeg

⅛ teaspoon ground ginger

8 slices Udi's gluten-free sandwich bread

1. Heat a large nonstick skillet over medium-high heat.

2. In a large bowl, whisk the eggs, rice milk, orange zest, stevia, cinnamon, nutmeg, and ginger. Pour the mixture into a 9-by-13-inch pan.

3. Add the bread to the custard and soak for 3 minutes.

4. Working in batches, add the soaked bread slices to the hot skillet and cook for about 4 minutes per side until the custard sets and the toast is browned.

for **PLAN A** Replace the 6 whole eggs with 8 egg whites and 2 whole eggs. Eliminate the cinnamon and increase the ground ginger to ½ teaspoon. Reduce the serving size by half or eat 1 full serving in 2 meals, 2 to 3 hours apart, to avoid overfilling your stomach.

for **PLAN C** Use a whole-grain gluten-free bread (such as Udi's whole-grain) in place of the sandwich bread for additional fiber.

BIG 8 ALLERGENS Replace the eggs with flaxseed eggs (see page 28).

PER SERVING Calories: 204; Total fat: 8g; Saturated fat: 2g; Carbohydrates: 22g; Fiber: <1g; Protein: 10g

BACON AND POTATO FRITTATA

PORTABLE Bacon makes virtually anything taste better, and the great thing about this smoky meat is you don't need a lot for a big flavor payoff. Aside from the smoky bacon flavor, this tasty frittata is a very satisfying way to eat a high-protein breakfast that keeps you going throughout the day. *Serves 4*

PREP 10 minutes
COOK 13 to 15 minutes

6 large eggs, beaten

¼ cup unsweetened rice milk

¼ teaspoon sea salt

⅛ teaspoon freshly ground black pepper

1 potato, peeled and grated

3 bacon slices, chopped

2 tablespoons grated Parmesan cheese

1. Preheat the broiler to high.

2. In a large bowl, whisk the eggs, rice milk, sea salt, and pepper.

3. Fold in the potato.

4. In a large ovenproof skillet over medium-high heat, brown the bacon for about 5 minutes until crisp.

5. Add the egg and potato mixture and cook for about 5 minutes more until the frittata sets around the sides. Sprinkle the Parmesan cheese over the top and transfer the skillet to the broiler.

6. Broil for 3 to 5 minutes until brown and puffed on top. Cut into slices and serve.

for **PLAN A** Replace the bacon with turkey bacon or Canadian bacon because it's leaner. Eliminate the Parmesan cheese and black pepper. Replace the 6 whole eggs with 6 egg whites and 2 whole eggs. Reduce the serving size by half or eat 1 full serving in 2 meals, 2 to 3 hours apart, to avoid overfilling your stomach.

for **PLAN C** Don't peel the potato before grating it. The peel adds fiber.

for **PLAN D** Eliminate the Parmesan cheese.

BIG 8 ALLERGENS If you are allergic to eggs, there isn't a replacement for eggs here, so avoid this recipe.

PER SERVING Calories: 266; Total fat: 17g; Saturated fat: 6g; Carbohydrates: 8g; Fiber: 1g; Protein: 19g

POTATO HASH WITH FRIED EGG

ONE-POT | **VEGETARIAN** When you put an over-easy egg on top of crunchy potato hash the result is absolute magic. The yolk runs down and coats the hash, adding yumminess to the crispy potato. Chives and thyme add even more flavor to this dish, which is just as easy to cook for one person as it is to cook for a whole family. *Serves 2*

PREP 5 minutes
COOK 20 minutes

2 tablespoons butter, divided

1 potato, peeled and cut into ½-inch cubes

2 tablespoons chopped fresh chives

½ teaspoon dried thyme

½ teaspoon sea salt, plus more for the eggs

⅛ teaspoon freshly ground black pepper

2 large eggs

1. In a large skillet or sauté pan over medium-high heat, melt 1 tablespoon of butter until it bubbles.

2. Add the potato and cook for about 10 minutes, stirring occasionally, until crisp and browned.

3. Stir in the chives, thyme, sea salt, and pepper. Cook, stirring, for 3 minutes more. Remove the potato from the pan and set aside.

4. Return the skillet to the heat and add the remaining 1 tablespoon of butter to melt, swirling the skillet to coat it.

5. Carefully crack the eggs into the skillet. Season with a pinch of sea salt. Cook the eggs for about 4 minutes until the whites are set. Flip the eggs. Turn off the heat and allow the eggs to sit for 30 seconds, just to warm the yolks. Place the eggs on top of the potato and serve.

for **PLAN A** Use nonstick cooking spray in place of the butter. Eliminate the black pepper.

for **PLAN C** Don't peel the potato before chopping it. The peel adds fiber.

for **PLAN D** Parboil the potato cubes for 5 minutes to soften before adding to the pan. Eliminate the chives.

BIG 8 ALLERGENS If you are allergic to eggs, there isn't a replacement for eggs here, so avoid this recipe.

PER SERVING Calories: 240; Total fat: 17g; Saturated fat: 9g; Carbohydrates: 16g; Fiber: 2g; Protein: 8g

ZUCCHINI, RED PEPPER, AND EGG SCRAMBLE

VEGETARIAN Not your average scrambled eggs here. Red bell peppers add a pop of color and a surprising sweetness to this simple breakfast scramble. You can make it vegan by replacing the eggs with 8 ounces of chopped tofu. This is a nutritious, easy-to-make meal that provides a hearty and satisfying high-protein breakfast. *Serves 4*

PREP 10 minutes
COOK 10 minutes

1 tablespoon extra-virgin olive oil

1 zucchini, chopped

1 red bell pepper, seeded and chopped

8 large eggs

2 tablespoons unsweetened rice milk

½ teaspoon sea salt

¼ teaspoon dried thyme

⅛ teaspoon freshly ground black pepper

1. In a large skillet or sauté pan over medium-high heat, heat the olive oil until it shimmers.

2. Add the zucchini and red bell pepper. Cook for 3 to 5 minutes, stirring occasionally, until the vegetables are soft.

3. In a medium bowl, whisk the eggs, rice milk, sea salt, thyme, and black pepper. Pour the eggs into the skillet over the vegetables. Cook for about 4 minutes, stirring occasionally, until the eggs are set.

for **PLAN A** Use nonstick cooking spray in place of the olive oil. Replace 4 of the eggs with 6 egg whites. Omit the red bell pepper and black pepper.

for **PLAN D** Omit the red bell pepper. Peel the zucchini before cooking it and sauté it for about 7 minutes until very soft before proceeding with the recipe.

BIG 8 ALLERGENS If you're allergic to eggs, omit the eggs and rice milk. Instead, add 8 ounces chopped tofu with the sea salt, thyme, and black pepper.

PER SERVING Calories: 190; Total fat: 14g; Saturated fat: 4g; Carbohydrates: 4g; Fiber: 1g; Protein: 14g

BELL PEPPER OMELET

VEGETARIAN Bell peppers and eggs are a classic combination. You'll love the sweetness that red bell peppers gain as they cook, while the green peppers add a hint of piquancy to the dish. This is a really simple omelet that makes a satisfying breakfast or dinner. It also reheats well, so be sure to save leftovers for another meal or a snack. *Serves 2*

PREP 10 minutes
COOK 15 minutes

1 tablespoon extra-virgin olive oil

½ red bell pepper, thinly sliced

½ green bell pepper, thinly sliced

¼ teaspoon sea salt

⅛ teaspoon freshly ground black pepper

4 large eggs, beaten

2 tablespoons unsweetened rice milk

1 ounce grated Swiss cheese

1. In a large skillet or sauté pan over medium-high heat, heat the olive oil until it shimmers.

2. Add the red bell pepper, green bell pepper, sea salt, and black pepper. Cook for about 5 minutes, stirring occasionally, until soft.

3. In a medium bowl, whisk the eggs and rice milk. Pour the egg mixture into the skillet over the peppers. Cook for 4 to 5 minutes without stirring until the eggs set around the edges. With a spatula, gently pull the edges away from the sides of the pan. Tilt the pan and allow the uncooked egg to run into the empty spaces. Continue cooking for 2 to 3 minutes more until the eggs are set.

4. Sprinkle the Swiss cheese on top of the eggs. Fold half of the omelet over onto itself, covering the cheese. Cook for 1 minute more.

for **PLAN A** Use nonstick cooking spray in place of the olive oil. Replace 2 of the eggs with 4 egg whites. Omit the red and green bell peppers and replace them with 1 sliced zucchini. Omit the cheese and black pepper.

for **PLAN D** Eliminate the green bell pepper and instead use 1 whole red bell pepper. Cook the pepper for about 7 minutes until very soft before proceeding with the recipe.

BIG 8 ALLERGENS If you're allergic to eggs, there's not really a way to make an egg-free omelet, so avoid this recipe.

PER SERVING Calories: 266; Total fat: 20g; Saturated fat: 6g; Carbohydrates: 7g; Fiber: 1g; Protein: 16g

HAM STRATA

MAKE AHEAD | PORTABLE A strata is a baked egg casserole that typically contains layers of meat, cheese, herbs, spices, and bread. It's an entire meal and it keeps very well, so you can make a batch and refrigerate it to reheat for meals on the go. Reheat it in the microwave for 1 to 2 minutes until hot. This makes a hearty breakfast, lunch, or dinner. *Serves 4*

PREP 10 minutes
COOK 1 hour

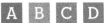

8 large eggs

¼ cup unsweetened rice milk

½ teaspoon dried thyme

½ teaspoon sea salt

¼ teaspoon freshly ground black pepper

6 ounces cooked ham, finely chopped

1 ounce grated Cheddar cheese

4 slices Udi's gluten-free sandwich bread, crusts removed and cut into cubes

Nonstick cooking spray, for the baking dish

1. In a large bowl, whisk the eggs, rice milk, thyme, sea salt, and pepper until well combined.

2. Stir in the ham, Cheddar cheese, and bread cubes. Refrigerate for 30 minutes.

3. Preheat the oven to 375°F.

4. Coat a 9-inch-square baking dish with cooking spray. Pour the strata mixture into the prepared pan. Bake for about 1 hour, or until set.

for **PLAN A** Replace 4 of the eggs with 8 egg whites. Eliminate the cheese and the pepper. Replace the ham with Canadian bacon, which is leaner. Reduce the serving size by half or eat 1 full serving in 2 meals, 2 to 3 hours apart, to avoid overfilling your stomach.

for **PLAN C** Replace the sandwich bread with Udi's whole-grain gluten-free bread for added fiber.

for **PLAN D** Eliminate the cheese if dairy causes you gastric upset.

BIG 8 ALLERGENS If you're allergic to eggs, there's not really a way to make an egg-free omelet, so avoid this recipe.

PER SERVING Calories: 256; Total fat: 15g; Saturated fat: 6g; Carbohydrates: 9g; Fiber: <1g; Protein: 21g

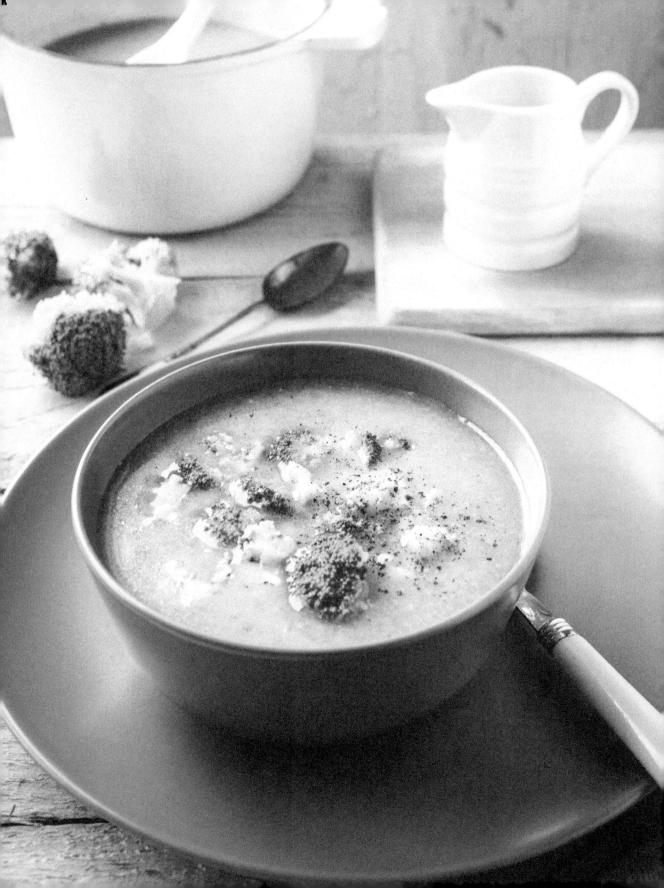

4

SOUPS AND SALADS

EASY TOMATO SOUP

MAKE AHEAD | **PORTABLE** | **VEGAN** Tomato soup is a favorite comfort food, and this easy version is packed with FODMAP-friendly flavors and ingredients. Using garlic oil adds a hint of garlic flavor, and finishing with fresh basil provides a bright herbal character that makes this soup extra tasty. This dish is a great make-ahead meal, so feel free to make a big batch and freeze it for convenient meals on busy days. *Serves 4*

PREP 10 minutes
COOK 15 minutes

1 tablespoon Garlic Oil (page 184)

3 scallions (green part only), chopped

2 tablespoons chopped fresh chives

2 (14-ounce) cans fire roasted tomatoes, undrained

2 cups Vegetable Broth (page 182)

½ teaspoon sea salt

¼ teaspoon freshly ground black pepper

3 tablespoons chopped fresh basil

1. In a large pot over medium-high heat, heat the garlic oil until it shimmers.

2. Add the scallions and chives and cook for 4 minutes, stirring occasionally.

3. Stir in the tomatoes, broth, sea salt, and pepper. Bring to a simmer, reduce the heat to medium-low, and cook for 10 minutes. Transfer the soup to a blender or food processor (or use an immersion blender). Blend until smooth and serve garnished with the fresh basil.

for **PLAN A** Tomatoes have a lot of acid, which can aggravate GERD. Avoid this recipe if you have IBS with GERD.

for **PLAN C** Stir ¼ cup cooked brown rice into each serving for additional fiber.

PER SERVING Calories: 89; Total fat: 5g; Saturated fat: <1g; Carbohydrates: 9g; Fiber: 3g; Protein: 4g

SAVORY VEGETABLE SOUP

MAKE AHEAD | ONE-POT | PORTABLE | VEGAN Vegetable soup makes a great meal because it's filled with healthy, nutritious veggies and you can choose any number and type to toss into the pot. It's easy to vary for all types of IBS and other symptoms. This soup freezes well and it's easily doubled or tripled for family meals. *Serves 4*

PREP 10 minutes
COOK 15 minutes

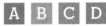

1 tablespoon Garlic Oil
(page 184)

3 scallions (green part
only), chopped

6 cups Vegetable Broth
(page 182)

2 carrots, peeled
and chopped

1 cup green beans, chopped

1 zucchini, peeled
and chopped

1 fennel bulb, chopped

1 teaspoon dried thyme

½ teaspoon sea salt

¼ teaspoon freshly ground
black pepper

1. In a large pot over medium-high heat, heat the garlic oil until it shimmers.

2. Add the scallions and cook for 3 to 4 minutes, stirring occasionally, until soft.

3. Stir in the vegetable broth, carrots, green beans, zucchini, fennel, thyme, sea salt, and pepper. Bring to a simmer, reduce the heat to medium-low, and cook for about 10 minutes, stirring occasionally, until the vegetables are soft.

for **PLAN A** Replace the garlic oil with 1 teaspoon extra-virgin olive oil. Eliminate the black pepper. Reduce the serving size by half or eat 1 full serving in 2 meals, 2 to 3 hours apart, to avoid overfilling your stomach.

for **PLAN C** Leave the peel on the zucchini and stir in 1 cup cooked quinoa just before serving, for added fiber.

for **PLAN D** Cook the vegetables for 10 to 15 minutes, or longer, until very soft. If garlic causes gastric upset, replace the garlic oil with extra-virgin olive oil.

PER SERVING Calories: 138; Total fat: 6g; Saturated fat: 1g; Carbohydrates: 13g; Fiber: 4g; Protein: 10g

CLAM CHOWDER

MAKE AHEAD | **ONE-POT** | **PORTABLE** Clam chowder typically has a dairy base, which makes it FODMAP-unfriendly. This version eliminates the dairy, replacing it with rice milk, but the flavor is still the traditional, smoky, creamy clam chowder you love. *Serves 4*

PREP 10 minutes
COOK 22 minutes

4 bacon slices, cut into small pieces

6 scallions (green part only), chopped

2 carrots, peeled and chopped

1 fennel bulb, finely chopped

1 red bell pepper, seeded and chopped

2 (6-ounce) cans chopped clams in clam juice, undrained

5 cups Poultry Broth (page 183)

1 teaspoon dried thyme

½ teaspoon sea salt

¼ teaspoon freshly ground black pepper

1 cup unsweetened rice milk

2 tablespoons cornstarch

1. In a large pot over medium-high heat, cook the bacon for about 5 minutes until it is browned. With a slotted spoon, transfer the bacon to a dish and set aside, leaving the grease in the pot.

2. To the pot, add the scallions, carrots, fennel, and red bell pepper. Cook for about 5 minutes, stirring occasionally, until the vegetables are soft.

3. Stir in the clams and their juice, broth, thyme, sea salt, and black pepper, using a spoon to scrape up any browned bits from the bottom of the pan. Bring to a simmer, reduce the heat to medium-low, and cook for 10 minutes, stirring occasionally. The vegetables should be very soft.

4. In a small bowl, whisk together the rice milk and cornstarch until smooth. Stir this slurry into the soup. Cook for about 2 minutes more, stirring constantly, until the chowder thickens.

5. Stir in the reserved bacon and serve.

for **PLAN A** Reduce the amount of bacon to 2 slices, or use 2 slices turkey bacon with 1 teaspoon extra-virgin olive oil. Eliminate the red bell peppers and black pepper. Reduce the serving size by half or eat 1 full serving in 2 meals, 2 to 3 hours apart, to avoid overfilling your stomach.

for **PLAN D** Test the red bell peppers for softness after about 10 minutes' cooking time. They should be very soft. Eliminate the scallions if the spiciness causes gastric upset.

BIG 8 ALLERGENS If you have an allergy to clams, make this chowder with chicken. Substitute 8 ounces cooked chicken breast for the clams and increase the amount of broth by 1 cup.

PER SERVING Calories: 363; Total fat: 15g; Saturated fat: 4g; Carbohydrates: 36g; Fiber: 4g; Protein: 20g

CHICKEN SOUP WITH ZUCCHINI NOODLES

MAKE AHEAD | ONE-POT | PORTABLE Chicken noodle soup can make just about anybody feel better. This version gets a low-FODMAP twist by replacing the traditional wheat-based noodles with zucchini noodles made with a spiralizer or julienne peeler. Or, use a vegetable peeler to cut the zucchini into ribbons and then a sharp knife to cut the ribbons into noodles. *Serves 4*

PREP 10 minutes
COOK 15 to 22 minutes

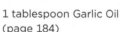

1 tablespoon Garlic Oil
(page 184)

12 ounces boneless skinless
chicken breast, cut into
½-inch pieces

3 carrots, peeled
and chopped

1 leek (green part only),
finely chopped

1 celery stalk, chopped

6 cups Poultry Broth
(page 183)

Juice of 1 lemon

Zest of 1 lemon

1 red bell pepper, seeded
and chopped

½ teaspoon dried rosemary

½ teaspoon sea salt

¼ teaspoon freshly ground
black pepper

Pinch red pepper flakes

1 medium zucchini, spiralized

1. In a large pot over medium-high heat, heat the garlic oil until it shimmers.

2. Add the chicken, carrots, leek, and celery. Cook for 5 to 7 minutes, stirring occasionally, until the chicken is cooked through.

3. Stir in the broth, lemon juice, lemon zest, red bell pepper, rosemary, sea salt, black pepper, and red pepper flakes. Bring to a simmer, reduce the heat to medium-low, and cook for 5 to 10 minutes, stirring occasionally, until the vegetables are soft.

4. Add the zucchini noodles and cook for 4 minutes more.

for **PLAN A** Eliminate the red bell peppers, black pepper, red pepper flakes, and lemon juice (retain the lemon zest). Replace the garlic oil with 1 teaspoon extra-virgin olive oil. Reduce the serving size by half or eat 1 full serving in 2 meals, 2 to 3 hours apart, to avoid overfilling your stomach.

for **PLAN D** Cut the chicken into smaller pieces so it becomes very soft as it cooks. Peel the zucchini before cutting it into noodles. If garlic causes gastric upset, replace the garlic oil with extra-virgin olive oil. You may wish to cook the soup for 2 to 4 minutes more after adding the zucchini noodles to ensure they are very soft.

PER SERVING Calories: 300; Total fat: 12g; Saturated fat: 3g; Carbohydrates: 13g; Fiber: 3g; Protein: 40g

MINESTRONE

MAKE AHEAD | **ONE-POT** | **PORTABLE** | **VEGAN** This rich Italian vegetable soup is loaded with hearty flavor and healthy vegetables. Typical minestrone includes kidney beans, which are high in FODMAPs. Instead, this recipe uses chickpeas. While chickpeas do contain FODMAPs, small amounts (about ¼ cup per person) won't trigger a flare-up. Be sure to use canned chickpeas—not fresh or dried—since FODMAP amounts vary. *Serves 4*

PREP 10 minutes
COOK 16 to 18 minutes

1 tablespoon Garlic Oil (page 184)

1 leek (green part only), chopped

1 celery stalk, chopped

1 fennel bulb, chopped

1 carrot, peeled and sliced

1 red bell pepper, seeded and chopped

6 cups Vegetable Broth (page 182)

1 zucchini, chopped

1 cup chopped green beans

1 cup canned chickpeas, rinsed and drained

1 (14-ounce) can crushed tomatoes, with juice

2 teaspoons dried Italian seasoning

1 teaspoon sea salt

¼ teaspoon freshly ground black pepper

2 tablespoons chopped fresh basil

1. In a large pot over medium-high heat, heat the garlic oil until it shimmers.

2. Add the leek, celery, fennel, carrot, and red bell pepper. Cook for 5 to 7 minutes, stirring occasionally, until the vegetables begin to brown.

3. Stir in the broth, zucchini, green beans, chickpeas, tomatoes with their juice, Italian seasoning, sea salt, and black pepper. Bring to a simmer, reduce the heat to medium-low, and cook for about 10 minutes, stirring occasionally, until the vegetables are soft.

4. Just before serving, stir in the basil.

for **PLAN A** Replace the garlic oil with 1 teaspoon extra-virgin olive oil. Eliminate the red bell peppers, crushed tomatoes, and black pepper. Increase the broth to 7 cups. Reduce the serving size by half or eat 1 full serving in 2 meals, 2 to 3 hours apart, to avoid overfilling your stomach.

for **PLAN D** If garlic causes gastric upset, replace the garlic oil with extra-virgin olive oil. Cut the vegetables into ¼-inch to ½-inch dice so they cook very well and are soft. Omit the chickpeas.

PER SERVING Calories: 283; Total fat: 8g; Saturated fat: 1g; Carbohydrates: 39g; Fiber: 12g; Protein: 17g

POTATO LEEK SOUP

MAKE AHEAD | ONE-POT | PORTABLE This soup is creamy and flavorful. While you can't use the white part of the leeks, here the green part is okay. Chop it finely so it softens quickly as you cook the soup. This simple soup is hearty and stores well in the refrigerator or freezer, so you can make a large batch for simple meals in a snap. *Serves 4*

PREP 10 minutes
COOK 20 to 25 minutes

3 bacon slices, cut into small pieces

2 leeks (green part only), thoroughly washed and finely chopped

2 tablespoons chopped fresh chives

6 cups Poultry Broth (page 183)

3 potatoes, peeled and cut into 1-inch pieces

1 teaspoon sea salt

¼ teaspoon freshly ground black pepper

1. In a large pot over medium-high heat, cook the bacon for 4 to 5 minutes, stirring occasionally, until browned. With a slotted spoon, remove the bacon to a dish and set aside, leaving the grease in the pot.

2. To the pot, add the leeks and chives. Cook for about 5 minutes, stirring occasionally, until the leeks are soft.

3. Stir in the broth, potatoes, sea salt, and pepper. Bring to a simmer, reduce the heat to medium-low, and cook for 10 to 15 minutes until the potatoes are soft. Transfer the soup to a blender or food processor (or use an immersion blender) and purée until smooth.

4. Serve the soup topped with the reserved bacon crumbles.

for **PLAN A** Reduce the amount of bacon to 1 slice and add 1 teaspoon extra-virgin olive. Use only 1 leek (green part only). Omit the black pepper. Reduce the serving size by half or eat 1 full serving in 2 meals, 2 to 3 hours apart, to avoid overfilling your stomach.

PER SERVING Calories: 311; Total fat: 11g; Saturated fat: 4g; Carbohydrates: 33g; Fiber: 5g; Protein: 19g

CREAM OF BROCCOLI POTATO SOUP

MAKE AHEAD | **ONE-POT** | **PORTABLE** This creamy, colorful soup makes a flavorful lunch or dinner. Easy to make ahead and refrigerate, you can simply heat it up on the stove top or in the microwave, which makes it perfect for a packed lunch. *Serves 4*

PREP 5 minutes
COOK 17 minutes

2 tablespoons Garlic Oil (page 184)

6 scallions (green part only), finely chopped

2 Russet potatoes, peeled and cut into 1-inch cubes

2 cups broccoli florets

6 cups Poultry Broth (page 183)

1 teaspoon dried thyme

½ teaspoon sea salt

¼ teaspoon freshly ground black pepper

1 cup unsweetened rice milk

2 tablespoons cornstarch

1. In a large pot over medium-high heat, heat the garlic oil until it shimmers.

2. Add the scallions and cook for about 4 minutes, stirring occasionally, until soft.

3. Stir in the potatoes, broccoli, broth, thyme, sea salt, and pepper. Bring to a simmer, reduce the heat to medium-low, and cook for about 10 minutes, stirring occasionally, until the potatoes are tender.

4. In a small bowl, whisk together the rice milk and cornstarch. Add this slurry to the soup in a thin stream, stirring constantly. Cook for about 2 minutes until the soup thickens.

for **PLAN A** Replace the garlic oil with 1 tablespoon extra-virgin olive oil. Eliminate the black pepper. Reduce the serving size by half or eat 1 full serving in 2 meals, 2 to 3 hours apart, to avoid overfilling your stomach.

for **PLAN D** Replace the garlic oil with extra-virgin olive oil. Purée the finished soup in a blender or food processor (or use an immersion blender).

PER SERVING Calories: 287; Total fat: 10g; Saturated fat: 2g; Carbohydrates: 38g; Fiber: 5g; Protein: 11g

GROUND BEEF AND VEGGIE SOUP

MAKE AHEAD | **ONE-POT** | **PORTABLE** Ground beef makes a great soup base, and cooking it in a single pot allows you to build lots of flavor. Feel free to experiment with your favorite low-FODMAP veggies here if you want to create some variation to this savory soup. For GERD, select the leanest ground beef you can find. *Serves 4*

PREP 10 minutes
COOK 20 minutes

12 ounces ground beef

1 teaspoon Garlic Oil
(page 184)

6 scallions (green part only),
finely chopped

2 carrots, peeled and sliced

1 red bell pepper, seeded
and chopped

1 medium zucchini, peeled
and chopped

6 cups Poultry Broth
(page 183)

2 cups shredded
green cabbage

1 teaspoon dried thyme

½ teaspoon ground
caraway seed

½ teaspoon dried
mustard powder

½ teaspoon sea salt

¼ teaspoon freshly ground
black pepper

1. In a large pot over medium-high heat, cook the ground beef in the garlic oil for about 5 minutes, crumbling it with the back of a spoon as you cook, until browned.

2. Add the scallions, carrots, red bell pepper, and zucchini. Cook for about 5 minutes more, stirring occasionally, until the vegetables soften.

3. Stir in the broth, cabbage, thyme, caraway, mustard powder, sea salt, and black pepper. Bring to a simmer, reduce the heat to medium-low, and cook for about 10 minutes until the vegetables are very soft.

for **PLAN A** Omit the garlic oil, cabbage, red bell pepper, and black pepper. Use the leanest ground beef you can find. Reduce the serving size by half or eat 1 full serving in 2 meals, 2 to 3 hours apart, to avoid overfilling your stomach.

for **PLAN D** Omit the cabbage. If garlic causes gastric upset, replace it with extra-virgin olive oil.

PER SERVING Calories: 270; Total fat: 9g; Saturated fat: 3g; Carbohydrates: 11g; Fiber: 3g; Protein: 35g

AMBROSIA SALAD

MAKE AHEAD | **ONE-POT** | **PORTABLE** | **VEGAN** The typical ambrosia salad is made with canned fruit cocktail and whipped cream. This version uses FODMAP-friendly fruits and coconut milk. It's a delicious side dish, and it also makes a tasty, healthy breakfast or snack. *Serves 4*

PREP 10 minutes
COOK 0 minutes

1 (14-ounce) can full-fat coconut milk, refrigerated overnight

Pinch ground nutmeg

1 cup hulled and chopped fresh strawberries

1 (14-ounce) can crushed pineapple in juice, drained

1 ripe banana, chopped

1 (11-ounce) can mandarin oranges in water, drained

1. Open the coconut milk and spoon the solid coconut cream on top into a large bowl. Discard the remaining coconut water.

2. Whisk the nutmeg into the coconut cream.

3. Add the strawberries, pineapple, banana, and mandarin oranges. Stir to coat the fruit with the coconut cream.

for **PLAN A** Replace the mandarin oranges with another banana. Replace the pineapple with 1 cup fresh blueberries. In place of the full-fat coconut milk, use ¼ cup canned light coconut milk whisked with the nutmeg. You don't need to refrigerate the light coconut milk overnight.

for **PLAN D** Omit the fresh strawberries and use only the canned pineapple, banana, and mandarin oranges.

PER SERVING Calories: 344; Total fat: 24g; Saturated fat: 21g; Carbohydrates: 35g; Fiber: 6g; Protein: 4g

KALE SALAD WITH FETA CHEESE AND WALNUTS

MAKE AHEAD | PORTABLE | VEGETARIAN Feta cheese and walnuts make a tasty flavor combination, particularly when used with basil vinaigrette and kale. This salad is simple to make, but if you do make it ahead of time, keep the salad and vinaigrette separate and toss them together just before serving. *Serves 4*

PREP 10 minutes
COOK 0 minutes

6 cups chopped kale, thoroughly washed and dried, stems removed, leaves torn into pieces

2 ounces crumbled feta cheese

1 cup chopped walnuts

½ recipe Basil Vinaigrette (page 185)

In a large bowl, toss the kale, feta, walnuts, and vinaigrette until combined.

for **PLAN A** Make the Basil Vinaigrette (page 185) using the GERD recipe substitutions and reduce the salad serving size by half or eat 1 full serving in 2 meals, 2 to 3 hours apart, to avoid overfilling your stomach.

for **PLAN D** This salad has too much texture and fiber for the IBD/IBS-D diet, so avoid it.

PER SERVING Calories: 462; Total fat: 43g; Saturated fat: 7g; Carbohydrates: 15g; Fiber: 4g; Protein: 14g

WARM SPINACH SALAD

Add a little cooked shrimp or chicken to this warm spinach salad, and you have a satisfying meal. It also makes a tasty side dish or a light meal on its own. This recipe calls for tender baby spinach, which wilts slightly when you add the delicious warm dressing. Don't be fooled by this salad's simplicity: it's wonderful. *Serves 4*

PREP 10 minutes
COOK 10 minutes

3 bacon slices, cut into small pieces

1 teaspoon Garlic Oil (page 184)

2 scallions (green part only), minced

¼ cup red wine vinegar

½ teaspoon sea salt

¼ teaspoon freshly ground black pepper

6 cups fresh baby spinach, thoroughly washed and dried

½ ounce grated Parmesan cheese

1. In a large skillet or sauté pan over medium-high heat, cook the bacon for about 5 minutes until crispy. With a slotted spoon, remove the bacon to a dish and set aside, leaving the grease in the pan.

2. To the pan, add the garlic oil, scallions, red wine vinegar, sea salt, and pepper. Simmer for about 5 minutes, stirring occasionally, until the scallions are soft.

3. In a large bowl, toss together the spinach, Parmesan cheese, and reserved bacon.

4. Pour the hot dressing over the spinach greens and toss to combine. Serve immediately.

for **PLAN A** Cook 1 bacon slice in 1 teaspoon extra-virgin olive oil instead of the garlic oil, then add the scallions, spinach, and sea salt. Sauté until cooked. Omit the black pepper, red wine vinegar, and Parmesan cheese. Reduce the salad serving size by half or eat 1 full serving in 2 meals, 2 to 3 hours apart, to avoid overfilling your stomach.

for **PLAN D** In step 2, add the spinach to the simmering vinaigrette. Cook until the spinach is soft—making cooked spinach instead of a salad. Omit the Parmesan cheese and sprinkle with the cooked bacon.

PER SERVING Calories: 153; Total fat: 11g; Saturated fat: 4g; Carbohydrates: 3g; Fiber: 1g; Protein: 10g

CHOPPED SALAD WITH BASIL VINAIGRETTE

MAKE AHEAD | **PORTABLE** Chopped salads make a great take-with meal, or a simple cold meal for a hot summer day. Using purchased rotisserie chicken makes the process super speedy. If you're taking the meal with you, don't toss the salad with the vinaigrette until just before you eat. *Serves 4*

PREP 10 minutes
COOK 0 minutes

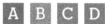

8 ounces cooked chicken breast, cut into ½-inch cubes

4 ounces cooked Canadian bacon, chopped

2 cups chopped iceberg lettuce

1 cup chopped black olives

½ cup canned drained and chopped artichoke hearts

8 cherry tomatoes, chopped

½ recipe Basil Vinaigrette (page 185)

2 tablespoons Mayonnaise (page 178)

Zest of ½ lemon

1. In a large bowl, toss together the chicken breast, Canadian bacon, lettuce, olives, artichoke hearts, and tomatoes.

2. In a small bowl, whisk together the basil vinaigrette, mayonnaise, and lemon zest. Pour the dressing over the salad and toss to combine.

for **PLAN A** Omit the cherry tomatoes. Reduce the olives to ½ cup and increase the lettuce to 4 cups. In place of the basil vinaigrette and mayonnaise dressing, mix ¼ cup very finely chopped fresh basil, the zest of ½ lemon, ¼ teaspoon sea salt, and ¼ cup plain coconut yogurt. Reduce the salad serving size by half or eat 1 full serving in 2 meals, 2 to 3 hours apart, to avoid overfilling your stomach.

for **PLAN D** Omit the lettuce, Canadian bacon, and cherry tomatoes. For a softer textured chicken, poach raw chicken cubes (12 ounces) in chicken broth for about 10 minutes until cooked.

PER SERVING Calories: 445; Total fat: 32g; Saturated fat: 5g; Carbohydrates: 17g; Fiber: 6g; Protein: 28g

CUCUMBER SALAD WITH ASIAN GINGER VINAIGRETTE

MAKE AHEAD | **PORTABLE** | **VEGAN** You'll love this zippy, refreshing cucumber salad with its sassy Asian flair. The cool cucumber flavor is the perfect match for the spicy ginger in the vinaigrette. If you're making this to go, mix the vinaigrette and salad just before you're ready to eat. *Serves 4*

PREP 10 minutes
COOK 0 minutes

2 medium cucumbers, peeled and chopped

½ recipe Asian Ginger Vinaigrette (page 186)

In a large bowl, toss together the cucumbers and vinaigrette.

for **PLAN A** Prepare the vinaigrette recipe using the GERD instructions (see page 186). Reduce the salad serving size by half or eat 1 full serving in 2 meals, 2 to 3 hours apart, to avoid overfilling your stomach.

for **PLAN D** This salad may have a little too much texture and spice. Try this recipe once your stomach has calmed a bit.

PER SERVING Calories: 195; Total fat: 20g; Saturated fat: 3g; Carbohydrates: 6g; Fiber: <1g; Protein: 1g

ROASTED VEGETABLE SALAD

MAKE AHEAD | **PORTABLE** | **VEGAN** Roasting the vegetables before dressing them makes this salad perfect for people with IBD/IBS-D who need softer food textures. Roasting not only alters the texture of the veggies, but also caramelizes them and adds tremendous savory flavor. You can serve this salad warm or cold. *Serves 4*

PREP 10 minutes
COOK 25 minutes

3 carrots, peeled and cut into ½-inch cubes

1 fennel bulb, cut into ½-inch cubes

1 medium zucchini, cut into ½-inch cubes

1 red bell pepper, seeded and chopped

2 tablespoons Garlic Oil (page 184)

½ teaspoon sea salt

¼ teaspoon freshly ground black pepper

Zest of ½ orange

½ recipe Basil Vinaigrette (page 185)

1. Preheat the oven to 450°F.

2. In a large bowl, toss the carrots, fennel, zucchini, red bell pepper, garlic oil, sea salt, black pepper, and orange zest until combined. Spread the vegetables on a baking sheet. Roast the vegetables for about 25 minutes until they begin to brown. Transfer to a large bowl.

3. Pour the vinaigrette over the warm roasted vegetables and toss to coat. Alternatively, let the vegetables cool completely and then toss them with the vinaigrette.

for **PLAN A** Omit the red bell pepper, garlic oil, black pepper, and basil vinaigrette. Instead, spray the vegetables with nonstick cooking spray before roasting, and for the dressing combine ¼ cup chopped fresh basil with ½ cup plain coconut yogurt and toss with the cooled vegetables. Reduce the salad serving size by half or eat 1 full serving in 2 meals, 2 to 3 hours apart, to avoid overfilling your stomach.

for **PLAN D** Replace the garlic oil with extra-virgin olive oil.

PER SERVING Calories: 297; Total fat: 28g; Saturated fat: 4g; Carbohydrates: 13g; Fiber: 4g; Protein: 2g

POTATO SALAD

MAKE AHEAD | PORTABLE | VEGETARIAN This potato salad is a riff on a loaded baked potato. This is a vegetarian dish, but if that's not a concern, add 4 slices crumbled, browned bacon to make it even tastier and to add a little protein. Keep this dish chilled until you're ready to serve. *Serves 4*

PREP 10 minutes
COOK 20 minutes

12 ounces small new red potatoes, halved

3 scallions (green part only), finely chopped

2 ounces Cheddar cheese, grated

2 tablespoons chopped fresh chives

½ cup plain coconut yogurt or lactose-free plain yogurt

½ teaspoon sea salt

¼ teaspoon freshly ground black pepper

1. In a large pot over high heat, combine the potatoes with enough water to cover and bring to a boil. Cook the potatoes for about 20 minutes until soft and then drain. Set aside to cool thoroughly.

2. In a large bowl, combine the cooled potatoes, scallions, Cheddar cheese, and chives.

3. In a small bowl, whisk the yogurt, sea salt, and pepper. Pour the dressing over the potatoes and gently toss to combine.

for **PLAN A** Omit the Cheddar cheese and black pepper. Use coconut yogurt and reduce the serving size by half or eat 1 full serving in 2 meals, 2 to 3 hours apart, to avoid overfilling your stomach.

for **PLAN D** Replace the unpeeled baby red potatoes with peeled white or Yukon Gold potatoes, cut into 1-inch cubes. Omit the Cheddar cheese.

PER SERVING Calories: 140; Total fat: 5g; Saturated fat: 3g; Carbohydrates: 16g; Fiber: 2g; Protein: 7g

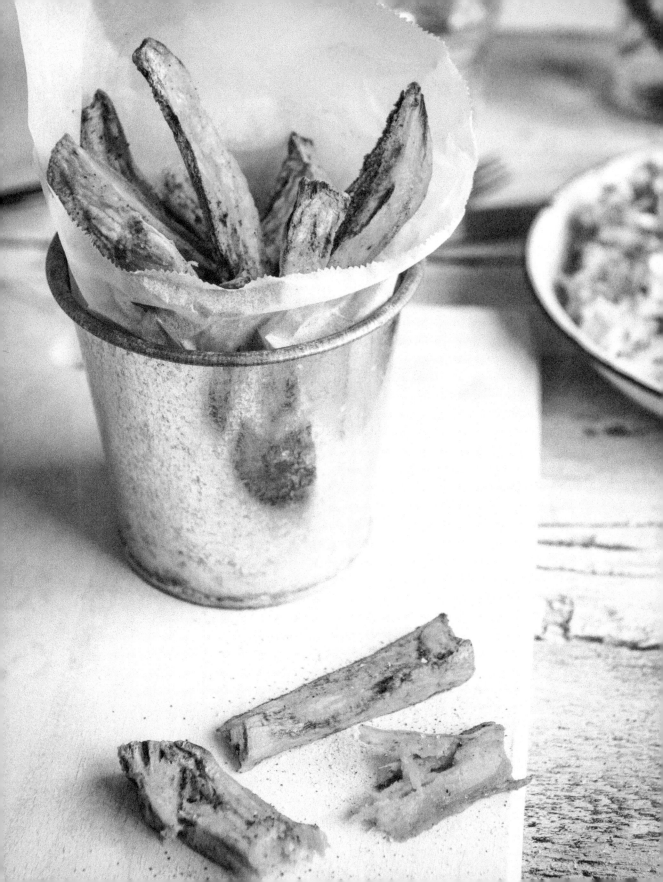

5

SNACKS AND SIDES

SPICED ROASTED PEPITAS

MAKE AHEAD | **PORTABLE** | **VEGAN** Pepitas are shelled pumpkin seeds. These tasty, tender seeds are good raw (and make a great FODMAP-friendly snack), and you can also dress up the flavor with all kinds of spices. This recipe uses a blend of Latin spices that complement the slightly sweet, earthy flavor of the pumpkin seeds. *Serves 8*

PREP 5 minutes
COOK 15 minutes

2 cups raw pepitas

2 teaspoons Garlic Oil (page 184)

½ teaspoon sea salt

½ teaspoon ground cumin

¼ teaspoon ground coriander

¼ teaspoon dried oregano

¼ teaspoon chili powder

1. Preheat the oven to 325°F.

2. Line a baking sheet with aluminum foil or parchment paper.

3. In a large bowl, toss together the pepitas, garlic oil, sea salt, cumin, coriander, oregano, and chili powder until combined. Spread the pepitas in a single layer in the prepared pan.

4. Bake for about 15 minutes, stirring occasionally, until the seeds are golden.

for **PLAN D** Texturally, these might be a bit rough for your stomach. If you have trouble with nuts and seeds, avoid this recipe. But you can make pumpkin seed butter by processing the pepitas in the food processor or blender with a little canola oil or extra-virgin olive oil. Enjoy it on gluten-free toast.

PER SERVING Calories: 198; Total fat: 17g; Saturated fat: 3g; Carbohydrates: 6g; Fiber: 1g; Protein: 9g

DEVILED EGGS

MAKE AHEAD | PORTABLE | VEGETARIAN One of the great things about deviled eggs is that once you have the basic formula down, the flavor possibilities are endless in the chopped herbs and spices you add to the yolk mixture. Keep the finished eggs chilled until you're ready to serve them. Slightly older eggs are easier to peel and work with than very fresh eggs. *Serves 6*

PREP 5 minutes
COOK 15 minutes

6 large eggs

¼ cup Mayonnaise (page 178)

2 tablespoons chopped fresh chives

2 tablespoons Dijon mustard

½ teaspoon sea salt

¼ teaspoon freshly ground black pepper

Paprika, for sprinkling

1. In a large pot over high heat, cover the eggs with cold water by about 1 inch. Bring to a boil. Turn off the heat. Cover the eggs and let them sit in the hot water for 14 minutes.

2. Plunge the eggs into a bowl of ice water to stop the cooking. Peel the eggs and halve them lengthwise.

3. With a small spoon, scoop the egg yolks into a small bowl and set the whites, cut-side up, on a plate.

4. To the yolks, add the mayonnaise, chives, Dijon mustard, sea salt, and pepper. Use a fork to mash the ingredients until well combined. Spoon the yolks back into the cavities of the egg whites.

5. Sprinkle with paprika.

for **PLAN A** Eliminate the black pepper and paprika. Replace the mayonnaise with an equal amount of unsweetened, fat-free, lactose-free plain yogurt or coconut yogurt.

PER SERVING Calories: 114; Total fat: 9g; Saturated fat: 2g; Carbohydrates: 3g; Fiber: 0g; Protein: 6g

SWEET AND SPICY PECANS

MAKE AHEAD | **PORTABLE** | **VEGETARIAN** Sweet and spicy is a crave-worthy flavor combination, and these pecans make it easy to satisfy that yen. They keep well, tightly sealed, for up to 2 weeks, so you can make a bigger batch (doubling the recipe) for plenty of healthy, handy snacks. *Serves 8*

PREP 5 minutes
COOK 20 minutes

2 cups raw pecan halves

¼ cup packed brown sugar

2 tablespoons unsalted butter, melted

1 teaspoon ground cinnamon

½ teaspoon sea salt

¼ teaspoon ground allspice

⅛ teaspoon cayenne pepper

1. Preheat the oven to 300°F.

2. Line a baking sheet with aluminum foil or parchment paper.

3. In a medium bowl, toss together the pecans, brown sugar, butter, cinnamon, sea salt, allspice, and cayenne pepper. Spread the seasoned nuts in a single layer in the prepared pan.

4. Bake for about 20 minutes until the nuts are golden. Cool completely before storing.

for **PLAN D** You'll know whether your stomach tolerates nuts, so use caution if you have difficulty with nuts and seeds. You can make nut butter by processing the pecans with 2 tablespoons of canola oil until smooth.

PER SERVING Calories: 241; Total fat: 23g; Saturated fat: 4g; Carbohydrates: 9g; Fiber: 3g; Protein: 3g

BAKED POTATO CHIPS

MAKE AHEAD | **PORTABLE** | **VEGAN** Commercial potato chips often contain questionable ingredients and are usually deep-fried so they're super fatty. It's easy to make your own baked potato chips, though, and you can make them with flavors you like, using the herbs and spices you have available. This recipe uses garlic oil, which imparts a subtle garlic flavor to the chips. *Serves 8*

PREP 15 minutes
COOK 30 minutes

3 medium potatoes, cut into ¼-inch-thick slices

3 tablespoons Garlic Oil (page 184)

1 teaspoon sea salt

1. Preheat the oven to 400°F.

2. Line two baking sheets with aluminum foil or parchment paper.

3. In a medium bowl, toss together the potatoes, garlic oil, and sea salt. Spread in the prepared pans in a single layer.

4. Bake for about 30 minutes until the potatoes are crisp and golden. Cool before storing.

for **PLAN A** Replace the garlic oil with 1 tablespoon extra-virgin olive oil.

for **PLAN D** You may wish to cook these potato chips to a softer consistency. You can do this by reducing the cooking time to just 20 minutes, or by cutting thicker slices. Also, if garlic upsets your stomach, peel the potatoes before slicing them and replace the garlic oil with extra-virgin olive oil.

PER SERVING Calories: 100; Total fat: 5g; Saturated fat: <1g; Carbohydrates: 13g; Fiber: 2g; Protein: 1g

SESAME KALE CHIPS

MAKE AHEAD | **PORTABLE** | **VEGAN** Kale is a superfood packed with antioxidants and nutrition. When cooked properly, you can make flavorful, delicately crispy kale chips that make a satisfying, healthy snack for your entire family. Store the kale chips in an airtight container in the cupboard for up to 2 weeks. *Serves 6*

PREP 10 minutes
COOK 1 hour

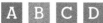

1 bunch kale, stems removed, leaves torn into bite-size pieces

¼ cup sesame seeds, white or black

2 tablespoons Garlic Oil (page 184)

¼ teaspoon sesame oil

Zest of 1 lemon

½ teaspoon sea salt

1. Preheat the oven to 200°F.

2. Line two baking sheets with aluminum foil or parchment paper.

3. In a medium bowl, toss together the kale, sesame seeds, garlic oil, sesame oil, lemon zest, and sea salt. Spread in the prepared pans in a single layer.

4. Bake for 30 minutes. Using a spatula, flip the kale. Continue cooking for about 25 minutes more until the chips are dried and crisp. Cool completely before storing.

for **PLAN A** Replace the garlic oil with ½ tablespoon extra-virgin olive oil.

for **PLAN D** Kale may be too harsh for IBD/IBS-D, so avoid this recipe.

PER SERVING Calories: 69; Total fat: 6g; Saturated fat: <1g; Carbohydrates: 4g; Fiber: <1g; Protein: 2g

ZUCCHINI HUMMUS

MAKE AHEAD | **PORTABLE** | **VEGAN** While canned chickpeas in small amounts are okay on low-FODMAP diets (less than ¼ cup per serving), if you have too many, it may make you uncomfortable. That's why this hummus dip uses a few chickpeas, but fills out the recipe with zucchini, which has a neutral flavor and a good texture for the dip. What you choose to dip into your hummus may depend on your IBS type. If you have IBD/IBS-D, choose a soft, low-FODMAP, gluten-free pita bread. For IBS-C, try red bell pepper slices. For GERD, dip carrots. While tahini is low in FODMAPS, limit your serving of this hummus to ¼ cup per day. *Serves 6*

PREP 10 minutes
COOK 0 minutes

½ cup canned chickpeas, rinsed and drained

2 tablespoons Garlic Oil (page 184)

1 zucchini, peeled and chopped

2 tablespoons tahini (sesame seed paste)

Juice of 1 lemon

Zest of 1 lemon

½ teaspoon sea salt

In a blender or food processor, combine the chickpeas, garlic oil, zucchini, tahini, lemon juice, lemon zest, and sea salt. Process until smooth.

for **PLAN A** Replace the garlic oil with ½ tablespoon extra-virgin olive oil. Omit the lemon juice and replace it with 2 tablespoons water.

for **PLAN D** If garlic upsets your stomach, replace the garlic oil with extra-virgin olive oil.

PER SERVING Calories: 103; Total fat: 6g; Saturated fat: <1g; Carbohydrates: 9g; Fiber: 3g; Protein: 3g

BAKED GREEN BEAN "FRIES"

PORTABLE | VEGETARIAN These "fries" are good either hot or cold. Make a dipping sauce with mayonnaise and herb/spice blends or eat as is. Either way, it's a delicious, nutritious, and easy-to-make low-FODMAP snack. *Serves 4*

PREP 10 minutes
COOK 15 minutes

2 slices Udi's gluten-free sandwich bread, processed into bread crumbs

1 teaspoon dried thyme

½ teaspoon sea salt

¼ teaspoon freshly ground black pepper

2 large eggs, beaten

2 tablespoons Garlic Oil (page 184)

1 pound fresh green beans, trimmed

1. Preheat the oven to 425°F.

2. Line a baking sheet with aluminum foil.

3. In a medium shallow bowl, mix the bread crumbs, thyme, sea salt, and pepper.

4. In a small shallow bowl, whisk the eggs and garlic oil.

5. Dip the beans into the eggs and then into the bread crumb mixture. Put in a single layer in the prepared pan.

6. Bake for 10 minutes. Using a spatula, flip the beans and then bake for 5 minutes more, or until crisp.

for **PLAN A** Omit the garlic oil and black pepper.

for **PLAN D** If garlic upsets your stomach, replace the garlic oil with extra-virgin olive oil.

BIG 8 ALLERGENS Replace the eggs with flaxseed eggs (see page 28).

PER SERVING Calories: 86; Total fat: 3g; Saturated fat: <1g; Carbohydrates: 12g; Fiber: 4g; Protein: 6g

GARLIC PARMESAN FRIES

PORTABLE | **VEGETARIAN** These simple oven fries are best hot, although in a pinch you can reheat them in the oven or microwave. Serve them with Barbecue Ranch Sauce (page 181) or Ketchup (page 179) for dipping. *Serves 4*

PREP 5 minutes
COOK 35 minutes

2 Russet potatoes, cut into ½-inch-wide strips

2 tablespoons Garlic Oil (page 184)

½ teaspoon sea salt

1 ounce Parmesan cheese, grated (optional)

1. Preheat the oven to 425°F.

2. Line a baking sheet with aluminum foil.

3. In a large bowl, toss the potatoes with the garlic oil, sea salt, and Parmesan cheese. Spread in a single layer in the prepared pan.

4. Bake for about 35 minutes until the potatoes are tender.

for **PLAN A** Replace the garlic oil with 1 tablespoon extra-virgin olive oil. Eliminate the Parmesan cheese.

for **PLAN D** Replace the garlic oil with extra-virgin olive oil and eliminate the Parmesan cheese.

PER SERVING Calories: 133; Total fat: 7g; Saturated fat: 1g; Carbohydrates: 17g; Fiber: 3g; Protein: 2g

YOGURT WITH FLAXSEED AND BLUEBERRIES

MAKE AHEAD | **PORTABLE** | **VEGETARIAN** Fruit and plain yogurt make a simple yet filling snack. You can use lactose-free plain yogurt or coconut plain yogurt, depending on what you have available. *Serves 1*

PREP 5 minutes
COOK 0 minutes

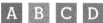

1 cup plain
unsweetened coconut or
lactose-free yogurt

1 tablespoon flaxseed

¼ cup fresh blueberries

In a small bowl, stir together the yogurt, flaxseed, and blueberries.

for **PLAN D** Omit the flaxseed. Cook the blueberries in a small saucepan with 2 tablespoons water for about 5 minutes until soft. You can also blend the blueberries and yogurt in a blender for a smooth texture.

BIG 8 ALLERGENS If you are allergic to dairy, use coconut yogurt.

PER SERVING Calories: 232; Total fat: 5g; Saturated fat: 3g; Carbohydrates: 25g; Fiber: 3g; Protein: 16g

BAKED ZUCCHINI CHIPS

MAKE AHEAD | **PORTABLE** | **VEGETARIAN** Zucchini chips make a healthy alternative to potato chips, and they are great if you're trying to watch carbs but still want something crispy. With their neutral flavor, these chips will take any type of seasonings you like. These are garlic and Parmesan, but you can get creative with your preferred herbs and spices. *Serves 4*

PREP 10 minutes
COOK 15 minutes

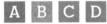

3 zucchini, cut into
¼-inch-thick slices

2 tablespoons Garlic Oil
(page 184)

2 tablespoons grated
Parmesan cheese

1. Preheat the oven to 350°F.

2. Line a baking sheet with parchment paper.

3. In a medium bowl, toss the zucchini slices with the garlic oil and Parmesan cheese. Place in a single layer in the prepared pan.

4. Bake for about 15 minutes until the cheese browns.

for **PLAN A** Replace the garlic oil with 1 tablespoon extra-virgin olive oil. Reduce the Parmesan cheese to 1 tablespoon.

for **PLAN D** Peel the zucchini before slicing. If garlic upsets your stomach, replace the garlic oil with extra-virgin olive oil. Eliminate the cheese and sprinkle the zucchini with ½ teaspoon sea salt.

BIG 8 ALLERGENS If you are allergic to dairy, omit the Parmesan cheese.

PER SERVING Calories: 95; Total fat: 8g; Saturated fat: 1g; Carbohydrates: 5g; Fiber: 2g; Protein: 3g

BLUEBERRY MUFFINS

MAKE AHEAD | **PORTABLE** | **VEGETARIAN** Blueberry muffins are so berry tasty, and they make a handy breakfast, snack, or side dish. These have a lovely cinnamon topping that makes them fragrant and delicious—you may have to fight your family to get your share.
Makes 12 muffins

PREP 10 minutes
COOK 12 minutes

   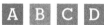

2 cups King Arthur gluten-free flour

2 teaspoons gluten-free baking powder

¾ cup sugar, divided

2 large eggs

1¼ cups unsweetened plain coconut yogurt, or lactose-free yogurt

⅓ cup canola oil

1 teaspoon vanilla extract

Zest of ½ orange

1 cup fresh blueberries

¼ cup melted unsalted butter

2 tablespoons ground cinnamon

1. Preheat the oven to 350°F.

2. Line a 12-cup muffin tin with paper liners.

3. In a large bowl, sift together the flour, baking powder, and ½ cup of sugar.

4. In a medium bowl, whisk the eggs, yogurt, canola oil, vanilla, and orange zest. Add the egg mixture to the flour mixture, and mix until just combined. Gently stir in the blueberries. Spoon the batter into the prepared muffin tin.

5. Bake for about 12 minutes until the muffins are cooked through. Cool them on a wire rack until still warm.

6. Put the melted butter in a small bowl.

7. In another small bowl, whisk together the remaining ¼ cup of sugar and the cinnamon.

8. Dip the top of each muffin in the melted butter and then in the cinnamon-sugar mixture.

for **PLAN A** Eliminate the cinnamon-sugar topping.

for **PLAN D** If dairy upsets your stomach, replace the melted butter with melted coconut oil or omit the cinnamon-sugar topping.

BIG 8 ALLERGENS If you are allergic to dairy, replace the butter with melted coconut oil.

PER SERVING Calories: 242; Total fat: 10g; Saturated fat: 6g; Carbohydrates: 33g; Fiber: 2g; Protein: 5g

GARLICKY GREEN BEANS AND RED BELL PEPPERS

MAKE AHEAD | PORTABLE | VEGAN This versatile side dish will add bright colors to your plate. The sweetness of the red bell peppers offsets the herbal flavor of the beans and the piquant garlic. Blanching the beans ahead of time allows them to cook quickly once they hit the pan. *Serves 4*

PREP 15 minutes
COOK 7 minutes

1 pound green beans, trimmed

2 tablespoons Garlic Oil (page 184)

1 red bell pepper, seeded and sliced

½ teaspoon sea salt

⅛ teaspoon freshly ground black pepper

1. Bring a large pot of water to a boil over high heat. Add the green beans. Cook for 1 minute, drain, then plunge the beans into a large bowl of ice water to stop the cooking. Drain again and set them aside.

2. In a large skillet or sauté pan over medium-high heat, heat the garlic oil until it shimmers.

3. Add the red bell pepper, green beans, sea salt, and black pepper. Cook for about 5 minutes, stirring occasionally, until the bell peppers are soft.

for **PLAN A** Eliminate the red bell pepper and black pepper. Replace the garlic oil with 1 tablespoon extra-virgin olive oil.

for **PLAN D** Instead of blanching the beans, boil them for about 5 minutes until tender, and drain thoroughly. While the green beans cook, sauté the red bell pepper in the garlic oil to soften it, and then add the cooked green beans and sauté for 3 to 5 minutes more until the vegetables are cooked to your desired tenderness. If garlic upsets your stomach, replace the garlic oil with extra-virgin olive oil.

PER SERVING Calories: 105; Total fat: 7g; Saturated fat: <1g; Carbohydrates: 10g; Fiber: 5g; Protein: 2g

CHIPS AND SALSA

MAKE AHEAD | PORTABLE | VEGETARIAN Corn chips are low in FODMAPs because they are made with field corn, not sweet corn, so they have a lower sugar level. It's easy to make your own chips using corn tortillas. And because you bake them yourself, there won't be any surprise ingredients. You can also use this fresh salsa to top fish or chicken, or as a delicious veggie dip. *Serves 4*

PREP 10 minutes
COOK 10 minutes

FOR THE CHIPS
4 corn tortillas, cut into wedges

1 tablespoon Garlic Oil (page 184)

½ teaspoon sea salt

FOR THE SALSA
2 large tomatoes, chopped

3 scallions (green part only), finely chopped

2 tablespoons chopped fresh cilantro

1 tablespoon Garlic Oil (page 184)

Juice of 1 lime

½ teaspoon sea salt

¼ teaspoon ground cumin

Pinch cayenne pepper

TO MAKE THE CHIPS

1. Preheat the oven to 400°F.

2. Line a baking sheet with parchment paper.

3. Brush the tortilla wedges with the garlic oil and put in the prepared pan in a single layer. Sprinkle with the sea salt.

4. Bake for about 10 minutes until crisp.

TO MAKE THE SALSA

1. In a medium bowl, combine the tomatoes, scallions, cilantro, garlic oil, lime juice, sea salt, cumin, and cayenne pepper.

2. Serve the chips with the salsa for dipping.

for **PLAN A** Salsa is not GERD-friendly, so avoid this recipe.

for **PLAN D** This may be a little bit too much roughage for you right now, but hold on to the recipe for when you feel better.

PER SERVING Calories: 133; Total fat: 8g; Saturated fat: 1g; Carbohydrates: 15g; Fiber: 3g; Protein: 2g

LOADED SMASHED POTATOES

MAKE AHEAD | PORTABLE Smashed red potatoes are a tempting dish all by themselves, but when you load them with bacon, chives, and cheese, you take them to a transcendent level. These potatoes are so good, this recipe is sure to be one you'll soon know by heart. *Serves 4*

PREP 15 minutes
COOK 15 minutes

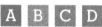

1 pound small new red potatoes, scrubbed

¼ cup unsweetened rice milk

3 bacon slices, browned, drained, and crumbled

1 ounce Cheddar cheese, grated

2 tablespoons chopped fresh chives

¼ cup plain lactose-free yogurt, or coconut yogurt

1 teaspoon sea salt

¼ teaspoon freshly ground black pepper

1. In a large pot over high heat, cover the potatoes with water and bring to a boil. Cook the potatoes for about 15 minutes until soft. Drain the potatoes and return them to the pot.

2. With a potato masher, smash the potatoes until they are smashed but still slightly chunky.

3. Stir in the rice milk, bacon, Cheddar cheese, chives, yogurt, sea salt, and pepper. Mix well.

for **PLAN A** Reduce the bacon to 2 slices and use turkey bacon instead. Omit the Cheddar cheese and black pepper. Reduce the serving size by half or eat 1 full serving in 2 meals, 2 to 3 hours apart, to avoid overfilling your stomach.

for **PLAN D** Use peeled potatoes to reduce the fiber content. Eliminate the Cheddar cheese. Whip the potatoes with an electric mixer until smooth if you need a softer or smoother texture.

BIG 8 ALLERGENS Replace the Cheddar cheese with hemp cheese.

PER SERVING Calories: 235; Total fat: 12g; Saturated fat: 5g; Carbohydrates: 21g; Fiber: 3g; Protein: 13g

MAPLE CORN BREAD

MAKE AHEAD | PORTABLE | VEGAN Corn bread can do triple duty as an appetizer, snack, or side dish. This corn bread is flavored with maple, so it has a lovely sweetness without using high-fructose honey, which is the typical corn bread ingredient. You can also bake this batter into muffins, but reduce the cooking time to about 18 minutes. *Serves 8*

PREP 10 minutes
COOK 25 minutes

Nonstick cooking spray, for the pan

1¼ cups King Arthur gluten-free flour

¾ cup cornmeal

2 teaspoons gluten-free baking powder

½ teaspoon sea salt

1 cup unsweetened rice milk

¼ cup pure maple syrup

¼ cup canola oil

1 tablespoon cornstarch

1. Preheat the oven to 400°F.

2. Coat an 8-inch-square baking pan with cooking spray.

3. In a large bowl, mix the flour, cornmeal, baking powder, and sea salt.

4. In a medium bowl, whisk the rice milk, maple syrup, canola oil, and cornstarch. Add the milk mixture to the flour mixture, and stir until just combined. Pour the batter into the prepared pan.

5. Bake for about 25 minutes until golden.

for **PLAN A** Reduce the serving size by half or eat 1 full serving in 2 meals, 2 to 3 hours apart, to avoid overfilling your stomach.

PER SERVING Calories: 217; Total fat: 8g; Saturated fat: 6g; Carbohydrates: 35g; Fiber: 1g; Protein: 3g

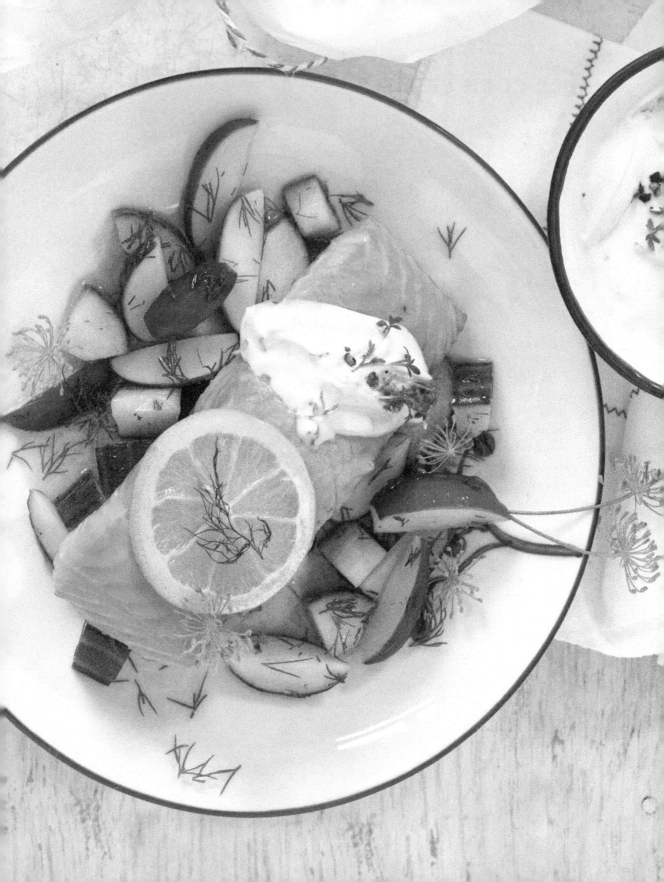

6

FISH AND SEAFOOD

SHRIMP AND GRITS

This southern classic is traditional comfort food for good reason. The creamy, cheesy grits are flavorful while the tender shrimp lends a sweet saltiness to the dish. This recipe calls for stoneground grits, but you can use quick grits, which will cook more quickly. Adjust cooking times according to the package instructions. *Serves 4*

PREP 10 minutes
COOK 30 to 35 minutes

4 cups water

1 teaspoon sea salt, divided

1 cup stoneground grits

1 tablespoon Garlic Oil (page 184)

2 ounces Cheddar cheese, grated

3 bacon slices, cut into small pieces

12 ounces shrimp, peeled, deveined, and tails removed

Juice of 1 lemon

Zest of 1 lemon

⅛ teaspoon freshly ground black pepper

2 tablespoons chopped fresh parsley

1. In a large pot over high heat, bring the water and ½ teaspoon of sea salt to a boil.

2. Stir in the grits. Reduce the heat to low and cook for 20 to 25 minutes, stirring occasionally, until soft and thoroughly cooked.

3. Stir in the garlic oil and Cheddar cheese.

4. While the grits cook, in a large skillet or sauté pan over medium-high heat, cook the bacon for 4 to 5 minutes until brown.

5. Add the shrimp and cook 4 to 5 minutes more, stirring occasionally, until the shrimp are pink.

6. Add the lemon juice, lemon zest, pepper, and remaining ½ teaspoon of sea salt. Cook for 2 minutes. Stir in the parsley. Serve the shrimp spooned on top of the grits.

for **PLAN A** Eliminate the garlic oil, lemon juice, and pepper. Reduce the bacon to 2 slices. Reduce the serving size by half or eat 1 full serving in 2 meals, 2 to 3 hours apart, to avoid overfilling your stomach.

for **PLAN D** Reduce the bacon to 1 slice. Simmer the shrimp in broth for 3 to 4 minutes and then cut them into small pieces before adding to the cooked bacon. Eliminate the Cheddar cheese. If garlic upsets your stomach, replace the garlic oil with extra-virgin olive oil.

BIG 8 ALLERGENS If you're allergic to shellfish, replace the shrimp with cubed boneless skinless chicken breast.

PER SERVING Calories: 257; Total fat: 13g; Saturated fat: 5g; Carbohydrates: 8g; Fiber: 1g; Protein: 26g

SHRIMP FRIED RICE

MAKE AHEAD | **ONE-POT** | **PORTABLE** Purchasing cooked rice (or cooking rice ahead of time and freezing it in 1-cup servings) is a big time-saver for rice dishes like this shrimp fried rice. It's loaded with flavor and comes together quickly. You can also make it ahead and take it with you when you're on the go—skip the takeout. *Serves 4*

PREP 10 minutes
COOK 15 to 17 minutes

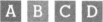

2 tablespoons Garlic Oil (page 184)

4 scallions (green part only), minced

1 carrot, peeled and cut into small cubes

1 teaspoon grated peeled fresh ginger

12 ounces shrimp, peeled, deveined, and tails removed

2 large eggs, beaten

4 cups cooked brown rice

2 tablespoons gluten-free soy sauce

1 tablespoon chopped fresh cilantro

1. In a large skillet or sauté pan over medium-high heat, heat the garlic oil until it shimmers.

2. Add the scallions, carrot, and ginger. Cook for about 5 minutes, stirring occasionally, until the carrot is soft.

3. Add the shrimp and cook for 3 to 4 minutes, stirring occasionally, until pink.

4. Add the eggs and cook for 2 minutes, stirring, until cooked through.

5. Stir in the rice and soy sauce. Cook for 4 to 5 minutes, stirring, until the rice is warm.

6. Sprinkle with the cilantro before serving.

for **PLAN A** Replace the garlic oil with 1 tablespoon extra-virgin olive oil. Reduce the serving size by half or eat 1 full serving in 2 meals, 2 to 3 hours apart, to avoid overfilling your stomach.

for **PLAN D** Simmer the shrimp and carrots in broth for about 5 minutes, or until soft, before adding them to the pan. Replace the brown rice with cooked white rice. If garlic upsets your stomach, replace the garlic oil with extra-virgin olive oil. Eliminate the fresh cilantro.

BIG 8 ALLERGENS If you are allergic to shellfish, replace the shrimp with an equal amount of boneless skinless chicken breast, tofu, or white fish.

PER SERVING Calories: 558; Total fat: 14g; Saturated fat: 3g; Carbohydrates: 77g; Fiber: 5g; Protein: 31g

SHRIMP SCAMPI WITH ZUCCHINI NOODLES

ONE-POT Zucchini noodles make a delicious base for this shrimp scampi, replacing traditional gluten-filled spaghetti noodles. In this recipe, make "zoodle" ribbons using a vegetable peeler or spiralizer to cut long, thin ribbons from the zucchini. *Serves 4*

PREP 10 minutes
COOK 15 minutes

2 tablespoons Garlic Oil
(page 184)

12 ounces shrimp, peeled, deveined, and tails removed

6 scallions (green part only), minced

½ teaspoon sea salt

1 cup dry white wine

1 cup Poultry Broth
(page 183)

Juice of 1 lemon

Zest of 1 lemon

2 zucchini, cut into noodle ribbons

⅛ teaspoon freshly ground black pepper

Pinch red pepper flakes

2 tablespoons chopped fresh flat-leaf parsley

1 ounce Parmesan cheese, grated

1. In a large skillet or sauté pan over medium-high heat, heat the garlic oil until it shimmers.

2. Add the shrimp, scallions, and sea salt. Cook for 4 to 5 minutes, stirring occasionally, until the shrimp is pink.

3. Stir in the white wine, broth, lemon juice, and lemon zest. Bring to a simmer and cook for 3 minutes more, stirring occasionally.

4. Add the zucchini, black pepper, and red pepper flakes. Cook 3 to 4 minutes, stirring occasionally, until the zucchini is al dente.

5. Garnish with the parsley and Parmesan cheese just before serving.

for **PLAN A** Replace the garlic oil with 1 tablespoon extra-virgin olive oil. Eliminate the lemon juice, black pepper, and red pepper flakes. Replace the white wine with an equal amount of broth. Reduce the Parmesan cheese to 2 table-spoons. Reduce the serving size by half or eat 1 full serving in 2 meals, 2 to 3 hours apart, to avoid overfilling your stomach.

for **PLAN D** Simmer the zucchini noodles in the broth in step 4 for 6 to 7 minutes until soft. If garlic upsets your stomach, replace the garlic oil with extra-virgin olive oil. Replace the white wine with an equal amount of broth.

BIG 8 ALLERGENS If you are allergic to shellfish, replace the shrimp with 12 ounces of cubed boneless skinless chicken breast or white fish of your choice.

PER SERVING Calories: 263; Total fat: 10g; Saturated fat: 3g; Carbohydrates: 8g; Fiber: 2g; Protein: 24g

LEMON PEPPER COD WITH ROASTED ROOT VEGETABLES

ONE-POT Cod is a flavorful, low-fat fish that cooks very quickly and tastes great with lemon and pepper. The roasted root vegetables add a touch of autumn to your plate and are an excellent source of vitamins and minerals. The result is a hearty dinner that's packed with flavor. *Serves 4*

PREP 10 minutes
COOK 35 to 40 minutes

2 carrots, peeled and roughly chopped

1 pound small new red potatoes, halved

2 turnips, peeled and roughly chopped

2 tablespoons extra-virgin olive oil, divided

1 teaspoon sea salt, divided

¼ teaspoon freshly ground black pepper, divided

1 pound cod, skin removed, cut into 4 pieces

Zest of 2 lemons

Juice of 2 lemons

1. Preheat the oven to 425°F.

2. In a large bowl, toss the carrots, potatoes, and turnips with 1 tablespoon of olive oil, ½ teaspoon of sea salt, and ⅛ teaspoon of pepper. Spread the vegetables in a single layer in a baking sheet and bake for 25 to 30 minutes until browned.

3. In a large skillet or sauté pan over medium-high heat, heat the remaining 1 tablespoon of olive oil until it shimmers.

4. Season the cod with the remaining ½ teaspoon of sea salt, ⅛ teaspoon of pepper, and the lemon zest.

5. Add the cod to the skillet and cook for 2 minutes.

6. Squeeze the lemon juice into the skillet with the oil, removing any seeds. Continue cooking for 2 minutes more. Flip the cod and cook for about 4 minutes more, or until the fish flakes easily with a fork.

for **PLAN A** Eliminate the black pepper and lemon juice. Add ¼ cup broth or water to the pan when you would add the lemon juice. Reduce the serving size by half or eat 1 full serving in 2 meals, 2 to 3 hours apart, to avoid overfilling your stomach.

for **PLAN D** Peel the potatoes. Instead of roasting the vegetables, simmer them in water or broth for 15 to 20 minutes until soft. Season them after cooking with sea salt and pepper (eliminate the olive oil). Poach the cod in the juice of 2 lemons and 2 cups broth for about 10 minutes, or until soft, instead of sautéing it. Season with sea salt and pepper after cooking.

BIG 8 ALLERGENS If you are allergic to fish, replace the cod with shrimp or use a thinly pounded boneless skinless chicken breast.

PER SERVING Calories: 291; Total fat: 8g; Saturated fat: 1g; Carbohydrates: 25g; Fiber: 5g; Protein: 29g

SIMPLE CRAB SALAD

MAKE AHEAD | PORTABLE Simple and sumptuous, this salad makes a delicious cold meal, and it's easy to pack for a portable lunch. When you work with precooked crab, it's important to pick it over to ensure there aren't shells in your finished salad. To do so, spread the crab on a platter and run your clean fingers through it, seeking any sharp pieces for removal. *Serves 4*

PREP 10 minutes
COOK 0 minutes

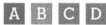

1 pound cooked lump crabmeat

3 scallions (green part only), finely chopped

½ cup finely chopped fennel bulb

⅓ cup Mayonnaise (page 178)

2 tablespoons chopped fresh fennel fronds

½ teaspoon sea salt

¼ teaspoon freshly ground black pepper

Zest of 1 lemon

Juice of 1 lemon

1. In a large bowl, toss together the crab, scallions, and fennel.

2. In a small bowl, whisk together the mayonnaise, fennel fronds, sea salt, pepper, lemon zest, and lemon juice. Pour the dressing over the crab mixture and gently toss to combine.

for **PLAN A** Eliminate the black pepper and lemon juice. Reduce the serving size by half or eat 1 full serving in 2 meals, 2 to 3 hours apart, to avoid overfilling your stomach.

for **PLAN D** Eliminate the raw fennel. Instead, cook 2 carrots (peeled and diced) in boiling water until soft. Drain the carrots and add them to the salad in place of the fennel.

BIG 8 ALLERGENS If you are allergic to shellfish, substitute cooked chicken breast or whitefish for the crab.

PER SERVING Calories: 205; Total fat: 9g; Saturated fat: 1g; Carbohydrates: 8g; Fiber: 1g; Protein: 24g

STEAMER CLAMS WITH FENNEL IN BROTH

ONE-POT Steamer clams make for a quick, easy meal. You can also use mussels in this dish—pick your favorite. After the elimination phase of this diet, if you find you can tolerate sourdough bread, dip warm sourdough in the broth to soak up all that brothy goodness. *Serves 4*

PREP 10 minutes
COOK 10 minutes

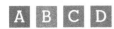

2 tablespoons unsalted butter

1 fennel bulb, chopped

6 scallions (green part only), chopped

5 pounds steamer clams in shells

1 cup dry white wine

Zest of 1 lemon

Juice of 1 lemon

2 cups Poultry Broth (page 183)

1 teaspoon dried tarragon

½ teaspoon sea salt

⅛ teaspoon freshly ground black pepper

1. In a large pot over medium-high heat, melt the butter until it bubbles.

2. Add the fennel and scallions. Cook for about 4 minutes, stirring occasionally, until the vegetables are soft.

3. Add the clams, white wine, lemon zest, lemon juice, broth, tarragon, sea salt, and pepper. Cover and cook for about 5 minutes until the clam shells open. Remove and discard any unopened clams before serving.

for **PLAN A** Reduce the butter to 1 tablespoon. Eliminate the black pepper and lemon juice. Reduce the serving size by half or eat 1 full serving in 2 meals, 2 to 3 hours apart, to avoid overfilling your stomach.

for **PLAN D** If your stomach is sensitive to dairy, replace the butter with extra-virgin olive oil.

BIG 8 ALLERGENS If you are allergic to shellfish, avoid this recipe. If you're allergic to dairy, replace the butter with extra-virgin olive oil.

PER SERVING Calories: 199; Total fat: 7g; Saturated fat: 4g; Carbohydrates: 20g; Fiber: 3g; Protein: 4g

VEGGIE-STUFFED TROUT

Stuffing trout with vegetables and herbs and baking it makes both the fish and the stuffing tender and flavorful. Feel free to experiment with vegetables and herbs you enjoy to make this recipe even more versatile. *Serves 8*

PREP 10 minutes
COOK 40 minutes

2 tablespoons Garlic Oil (page 184)

4 scallions (green part only), minced

2 carrots, peeled and minced

½ fennel bulb, peeled and minced

1 cup bread crumbs made from Udi's gluten-free sandwich bread

1 teaspoon sea salt, divided

¼ teaspoon freshly ground black pepper, divided

Zest of 1 lemon

Juice of 1 lemon

¼ cup Poultry Broth (page 183)

1 teaspoon dried dill

¼ cup chopped fresh flat-leaf parsley

4 (6- to 8-ounce) whole trout

1. Preheat the oven to 350°F.

2. In a large skillet or sauté pan over medium-high heat, heat the garlic oil until it shimmers.

3. Add the scallions, carrots, and fennel. Cook for about 5 minutes, stirring occasionally, until soft. Transfer the vegetables to a large bowl.

4. To the vegetables, add the bread crumbs, ½ teaspoon of sea salt, ⅛ teaspoon of pepper, the lemon zest, lemon juice, broth, dill, and parsley. Stir to combine.

5. If your trout isn't already cut down the middle and cleaned, cut them open, clean the cavity, and stuff the veggie–bread crumb mixture into it. Close the trout halves together. Place the trout in a baking dish and sprinkle the outside with the remaining ½ teaspoon of sea salt and ⅛ teaspoon of pepper.

6. Bake the trout for about 35 minutes until cooked through.

for **PLAN A** Replace the garlic oil with 1 tablespoon extra-virgin olive oil. Eliminate the lemon juice and replace it with 1 tablespoon broth. Eliminate the black pepper. Reduce the serving size by half or eat 1 full serving in 2 meals, 2 to 3 hours apart, to avoid overfilling your stomach.

for **PLAN D** If garlic upsets your stomach, replace the garlic oil with extra-virgin olive oil. Simmer the vegetables in 1 cup broth for 5 to 10 minutes until soft, instead of sautéing them. Stir the vegetables and broth into the bread crumb mixture. Cover the stuffed trout with aluminum foil and bake the trout covered so it steams and softens as it cooks.

BIG 8 ALLERGENS If you are allergic to fish, avoid this recipe. Alternatively, you can pound 4 (6-ounce) boneless skinless chicken breasts very thin and wrap them around the stuffing. Cover with aluminum foil and bake for about 35 minutes.

PER SERVING Calories: 313; Total fat: 14g; Saturated fat: 2g; Carbohydrates: 13g; Fiber: 2g; Protein: 33g

PAN-SEARED SCALLOPS WITH ORANGE AIOLI

Scallops have a slightly sweet, delicate, briny flavor that goes well with this tasty orange aioli. When choosing scallops, select those without any fishy scent, which means they are fresh. You can also use frozen, thawed scallops. Serve this with the Warm Spinach Salad (page 89) for a complete meal. *Serves 4*

PREP 10 minutes
COOK 10 minutes

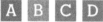

2 tablespoons
unsalted butter

1 pound sea scallops

½ teaspoon sea salt

¼ teaspoon freshly ground
black pepper

¼ cup Mayonnaise
(page 178)

2 tablespoons freshly
squeezed orange juice

1 teaspoon chopped
fresh tarragon

Zest of 1 orange

1. In a large skillet or sauté pan over medium-high heat, melt the butter until it bubbles.

2. Season the scallops with the sea salt and pepper and add them to the skillet. Sear the scallops in the hot butter for 2 to 3 minutes per side until browned.

3. In a small bowl, whisk the mayonnaise, orange juice, tarragon, and orange zest. Serve drizzled over the scallops.

for **PLAN A** Reduce the butter to 1 tablespoon. Eliminate the black pepper and orange juice. Reduce the serving size by half or eat 1 full serving in 2 meals, 2 to 3 hours apart, to avoid overfilling your stomach.

BIG 8 ALLERGENS If you are allergic to shellfish, avoid this recipe.

PER SERVING Calories: 212; Total fat: 12g; Saturated fat: 5g; Carbohydrates: 7g; Fiber: 0g; Protein: 19g

SALMON WITH DILL SAUCE AND RADISH SALAD

Serving simple baked salmon on a refreshing, crunchy salad makes a lovely light meal perfect for warm summer evenings. Dill plays a supporting role throughout this dish, flavoring the vinaigrette for the salad as well as the sauce for the salmon. *Serves 4*

PREP 5 minutes
COOK 15 minutes

FOR THE SALMON

4 (4- to 6-ounce) salmon steaks

½ teaspoon sea salt

⅛ teaspoon freshly ground black pepper

FOR THE DILL SAUCE

¼ cup Greek yogurt

1 tablespoon chopped fresh dill fronds

Zest of 1 lemon

¼ teaspoon sea salt

FOR THE SALAD

1 cup chopped red radishes

1 medium zucchini, chopped

2 tablespoons extra-virgin olive oil

1 tablespoon freshly squeezed lemon juice

1 teaspoon chopped fresh dill fronds

¼ teaspoon sea salt

Pinch freshly ground black pepper

TO MAKE THE SALMON

1. Preheat the oven to 425°F.

2. Line a baking sheet with aluminum foil.

3. Sprinkle the salmon with the sea salt and pepper and place in the prepared pan.

4. Bake for about 15 minutes until the salmon is opaque.

TO MAKE THE DILL SAUCE

In a small bowl, whisk together the yogurt, dill, lemon zest, and sea salt. Refrigerate until needed.

TO MAKE THE SALAD

1. In a medium bowl, combine the radishes and zucchini.

2. In a small bowl, whisk together the olive oil, lemon juice, dill, sea salt, and pepper. Pour the dressing over the vegetables and toss to coat.

3. Divide the salad among 4 plates, put a salmon steak on top of each salad, and spoon the dill sauce over the top.

for **PLAN A** Eliminate the black pepper. Reduce the serving size by half or eat 1 full serving in 2 meals, 2 to 3 hours apart, to avoid overfilling your stomach.

for **PLAN D** Eliminate the salad.

PER SERVING Calories: 315; Total fat: 18g; Saturated fat: 3g; Carbohydrates: 4g; Fiber: 1g; Protein: 36g

MAPLE-SOY GLAZED SALMON WITH TRI-PEPPER SAUTÉ

Baking salmon in a maple and soy glaze adds a delicate sweetness to this earthy fish. Salmon is an excellent source of omega-3 fatty acids, which are inflammation fighters, so this is a great recipe if you're also struggling with inflammation. *Serves 4*

PREP 15 minutes
COOK 25 minutes

¼ cup gluten-free soy sauce

¼ cup pure maple syrup

Zest of 1 orange

Juice of 1 orange

1 teaspoon grated peeled fresh ginger

4 (6-ounce) skin-on salmon fillets

2 tablespoons Garlic Oil (page 184)

1 red bell pepper, seeded and sliced

1 yellow bell pepper, seeded and sliced

1 orange bell pepper, seeded and sliced

½ teaspoon sea salt

⅛ teaspoon freshly ground black pepper

¼ cup dry white wine

1. Preheat the oven to 425°F.

2. In a large, shallow, rimmed dish, whisk the soy sauce, maple syrup, orange zest, orange juice, and ginger. Place the salmon in the dish skin-side up so the flesh marinates. Let it sit in the mixture for 10 minutes. Transfer the salmon, skin-side down, to a rimmed baking dish. Brush the marinade over the top of the salmon. Discard the remaining marinade.

3. Bake for 20 to 25 minutes until the salmon is opaque.

4. Meanwhile, in a large skillet or sauté pan over medium-high heat, heat the garlic oil until it shimmers.

5. Add the red, yellow, and orange bell peppers, salt, and black pepper. Cook for about 5 minutes, stirring occasionally, until the bell peppers are soft.

6. Stir in the white wine. Cover and cook for 5 minutes more. Serve the salmon on top of the bell peppers.

for **PLAN A** Replace the bell peppers with 2 fennel bulbs, thinly sliced. Replace the garlic oil with 1 tablespoon extra-virgin olive oil. Replace the white wine with an equal amount of broth. Eliminate the black pepper and orange juice (but use the orange zest). Reduce the serving size by half or eat 1 full serving in 2 meals, 2 to 3 hours apart, to avoid overfilling your stomach.

for **PLAN D** Cover the salmon with aluminum foil as it cooks so it steams lightly. Increase the liquid in the bell peppers to 1 cup by adding more water or broth. Cover and cook for 10 minutes to soften the bell peppers.

BIG 8 ALLERGENS If you are allergic to fish, replace the salmon with boneless skinless chicken breast. Reduce the oven temperature to 400°F and cook for 10 to 15 minutes, or until the chicken is done.

PER SERVING Calories: 393; Total fat: 18g; Saturated fat: 2g; Carbohydrates: 22g; Fiber: 2g; Protein: 35g

HEARTY FISH STEW

MAKE AHEAD | ONE-POT | PORTABLE This hearty fish stew is fragrant and savory with lively herbs and a delicate orange flavor. This dish comes together quickly and, with big chunks of vegetables and fish, it is warming and satisfying. *Serves 6*

PREP 10 minutes
COOK 25 minutes

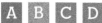

2 tablespoons extra-virgin olive oil

2 pounds boneless skinless white fish, cut into 1-inch chunks

1 fennel bulb, chopped

1 leek (green part only), chopped

16 small new red potatoes, halved

3 carrots, peeled and chopped

1 (14-ounce) can fire roasted tomatoes, undrained

4 cups Poultry Broth (page 183)

1 cup dry white wine

Zest of 1 orange

Juice of 1 orange

2 tablespoons chopped fresh fennel fronds

1 teaspoon dried tarragon

1 teaspoon dried thyme

1 teaspoon sea salt

¼ teaspoon freshly ground black pepper

2 tablespoons cornstarch

2 tablespoons water

2 tablespoons chopped fresh parsley

1. In a large pot over medium-high heat, heat the olive oil until it shimmers.

2. Add the fish, fennel, and leek. Cook for 5 minutes, stirring occasionally.

3. Add the potatoes, carrots, tomatoes, broth, wine, orange zest, orange juice, fennel fronds, tarragon, thyme, sea salt, and pepper. Stir to combine and bring to a simmer. Reduce the heat to low and cook for about 10 minutes, stirring occasionally, until the vegetables are very tender.

4. In a small bowl, whisk together the cornstarch and water. Stir this slurry into the stew. Cook for about 3 minutes, stirring constantly, until the stew thickens. Stir in the parsley and serve.

for **PLAN A** Eliminate the black pepper, tomatoes, and orange juice (use the orange zest), adding an additional cup of broth instead. Reduce the serving size by half or eat 1 full serving in 2 meals, 2 to 3 hours apart, to avoid overfilling your stomach.

for **PLAN D** Eliminate the fennel. Peel the potatoes. As the stew simmers, cover it to steam the vegetables and fish. Replace the white wine with an equal amount of broth.

BIG 8 ALLERGENS If you are allergic to fish, replace it with shrimp or cubed boneless skinless chicken breast.

PER SERVING Calories: 446; Total fat: 9g; Saturated fat: 2g; Carbohydrates: 33g; Fiber: 5g; Protein: 49g

FISH AND CHIPS

PORTABLE Classic fish and chips are breaded in a beer batter and deep-fried. You can still get the flavor and character of fish and chips minus the fat and all the high-FODMAP ingredients with just a few substitutions. If this dish is a particular favorite of yours, use this recipe and celebrate knowing there's no need to give it up. *Serves 4*

PREP 10 minutes
COOK 40 minutes

2 pounds potatoes, cut into wedges

2 tablespoons extra-virgin olive oil

1 teaspoon sea salt, divided

3 slices Udi's gluten-free sandwich, processed into bread crumbs

¼ cup cornmeal

2 tablespoons King Arthur gluten-free flour

½ teaspoon paprika

⅛ teaspoon freshly ground black pepper

1 large egg, beaten

1 tablespoon Dijon mustard

1 pound boneless skinless cod, cut into 1-inch pieces

1. Preheat the oven to 425°F.

2. In a large pot filled with boiling water, blanch the potato wedges for 5 minutes. Drain, pat dry, and transfer to a medium bowl.

3. Toss the potatoes with the olive oil and ½ teaspoon of sea salt and arrange them on a baking sheet. Bake, turning occasionally, for 35 minutes, or until tender.

4. In a large bowl, mix the remaining ½ teaspoon of sea salt, the bread crumbs, cornmeal, flour, paprika, and pepper.

5. In a large, shallow bowl, whisk the egg and mustard.

6. Dip the cod pieces into the egg mixture, then into the bread crumb mixture, and place on a second baking sheet. Add to the oven during the last 15 minutes of cooking time. Cook for about 15 minutes, until cooked through.

for **PLAN A** Eliminate the black pepper and paprika. Reduce the olive oil to 1 tablespoon. Reduce the serving size by half or eat 1 full serving in 2 meals, 2 to 3 hours apart, to avoid over-filling your stomach.

for **PLAN D** Peel the potatoes and blanch them for an additional 5 minutes. Replace the cornmeal with an additional ¼ cup gluten-free flour. Eliminate the paprika.

BIG 8 ALLERGENS If you are allergic to fish, replace it with boneless skinless chicken breasts cut into 1-inch pieces.

PER SERVING Calories: 503; Total fat: 11g; Saturated fat: 2g; Carbohydrates: 64g; Fiber: 8g; Protein: 36g

HALIBUT WITH RICE AND PINEAPPLE SALSA

MAKE AHEAD | **PORTABLE** The lively flavors in the rice and salsa give this fish dish a bright, vibrant taste that will remind you of a tropical vacation. It's a festive, tasty, and easy-to-prepare meal, especially when you use precooked rice, which will save you lots of time. You can find precooked rice in the rice section of your grocery store, or make your own ahead of time and freeze it in 1-cup servings. *Serves 4*

PREP 10 minutes
COOK 15 minutes

1 pound halibut fillet

2 tablespoons Garlic Oil (page 184)

½ teaspoon chili powder

1½ teaspoons sea salt, divided

⅛ teaspoon freshly ground black pepper

Zest of 1 lime

2 cups cooked brown rice

1 cup canned full-fat coconut milk

2 cups canned crushed pineapple in juice, drained

6 scallions (green part only), minced

¼ cup chopped fresh cilantro

½ jalapeño pepper, seeded and finely minced

2 tablespoons freshly squeezed lime juice

1. Preheat the oven to 400°F.

2. Line a baking sheet with parchment paper.

3. Brush the halibut with the garlic oil and sprinkle it with the chili powder, ½ teaspoon of sea salt, the black pepper, and lime zest. Place the fish in the prepared baking sheet, skin-side down.

4. Bake for 12 to 15 minutes (or longer for a thick fillet) until the fish is cooked through.

5. In a medium pot over medium-high heat, stir together the rice, coconut milk, and ½ teaspoon of sea salt until warm.

6. In a medium bowl, mix the pineapple, scallions, cilantro, jalapeño, lime juice, and the remaining ½ teaspoon of sea salt.

7. To serve, mound the rice. Place the fish over the rice and top with the salsa.

for **PLAN A** Eliminate the chili powder, black pepper, and salsa. Reduce the serving size by half or eat 1 full serving in 2 meals, 2 to 3 hours apart, to avoid overfilling your stomach.

for **PLAN D** Eliminate the jalapeño. Cover the fish with aluminum foil so it will steam and soften as it cooks. Blend the salsa in a blender or food processor to make it more of a sauce. Replace the brown rice with white rice. If garlic upsets your stomach, replace the garlic oil with extra-virgin olive oil.

BIG 8 ALLERGENS If you are allergic to fish, replace the halibut with shrimp (bake it for about 10 minutes), or boneless skinless chicken breast (325°F, cooked for 10 to 15 minutes).

PER SERVING Calories: 539; Total fat: 24g; Saturated fat: 14g; Carbohydrates: 52g; Fiber: 5g; Protein: 32g

CINNAMON SHRIMP

MAKE AHEAD | **ONE-POT** | **PORTABLE** The flavor of cinnamon adds something special to these shrimp. You'll love this sweet, slightly spicy stir-fry because it comes together quickly and is very flavorful. It will keep in the refrigerator for up to 3 days, so it's also a great make-ahead meal you can reheat when you're on the go or need a delicious meal fast. *Serves 4*

PREP 10 minutes
COOK 20 minutes

2 tablespoons extra-virgin olive oil

6 scallions (green part only), minced

4 carrots, peeled and diced

1 pound shrimp, peeled, deveined, and tails removed

1 cup Poultry Broth (page 183)

2 tablespoons pure maple syrup

2 tablespoons gluten-free soy sauce

1 teaspoon ground cinnamon

½ teaspoon grated peeled fresh ginger

1½ cups cooked brown rice

1. In a large skillet or sauté pan over medium-high heat, heat the olive oil until it shimmers.

2. Add the scallions and carrots. Cook for 5 to 7 minutes, stirring occasionally, until the carrots are soft.

3. Add the shrimp. Cook for about 5 minutes, stirring occasionally, until the shrimp are opaque.

4. Stir in the broth, maple syrup, soy sauce, cinnamon, and ginger. Bring to a simmer, reduce the heat to medium-low, and cook for 3 minutes more.

5. Stir in the rice. Cook for 3 minutes more until the rice is just warmed.

for **PLAN A** Reduce the olive oil to 1 tablespoon. Replace the cinnamon with ½ teaspoon ground ginger. Reduce the serving size by half or eat 1 full serving in 2 meals, 2 to 3 hours apart, to avoid overfilling your stomach.

for **PLAN D** Boil the carrots in water or broth for 5 minutes before adding to the pot. Cover while cooking the shrimp. Replace the brown rice with white rice.

BIG 8 ALLERGENS If you are allergic to shellfish, replace it with a whitefish, such as halibut or cod, cut into cubes, or boneless skinless chicken breast.

PER SERVING Calories: 398; Total fat: 10g; Saturated fat: 2g; Carbohydrates: 45g; Fiber: 4g; Protein: 32g

FISH CURRY

MAKE AHEAD | ONE-POT | PORTABLE This delicious curry has a coconut base that gives it a creamy, exotic flavor. You can replace the cod with any white fish you enjoy or find available in your region, with similar flavor results. *Serves 6*

PREP 10 minutes
COOK 20 minutes

2 tablespoons Garlic Oil (page 184)

1 tablespoon curry powder

6 scallions (green part only), minced

2 carrots, peeled and roughly chopped

1 zucchini, roughly chopped

1½ pounds boneless skinless cod, cut into 1-inch pieces

2 cups Poultry Broth (page 183)

1 cup canned full-fat coconut milk

½ teaspoon sea salt

1½ cups cooked brown rice

1. In a large pot over medium-high heat, heat the garlic oil until it shimmers.

2. Add the curry powder and cook for 30 seconds, stirring constantly.

3. Add the scallions, carrots, and zucchini. Cook for about 5 minutes, stirring occasionally, until the vegetables are soft.

4. Stir in the cod, broth, coconut milk, and sea salt. Bring to a simmer. Reduce the heat to low, cover, and cook for 5 to 10 minutes until the fish is soft.

5. Stir in the brown rice and cook 3 minutes more to warm the rice.

for **PLAN A** Replace the garlic oil with 1 tablespoon extra-virgin olive oil. Use light coconut milk. Reduce the serving size by half or eat 1 full serving in 2 meals, 2 to 3 hours apart, to avoid overfilling your stomach.

for **PLAN D** If garlic upsets your stomach, replace the garlic oil with extra-virgin olive oil. For steps 3 and 4, add all the remaining ingredients (except the rice) to the pot, bring to a simmer, reduce the heat to low, cover, and cook for 10 minutes to soften the vegetables and the fish. Replace the brown rice with white rice.

BIG 8 ALLERGENS If you are allergic to fish, replace it with shrimp or boneless skinless chicken breast.

PER SERVING Calories: 452; Total fat: 16g; Saturated fat: 10g; Carbohydrates: 44g; Fiber: 3g; Protein: 33g

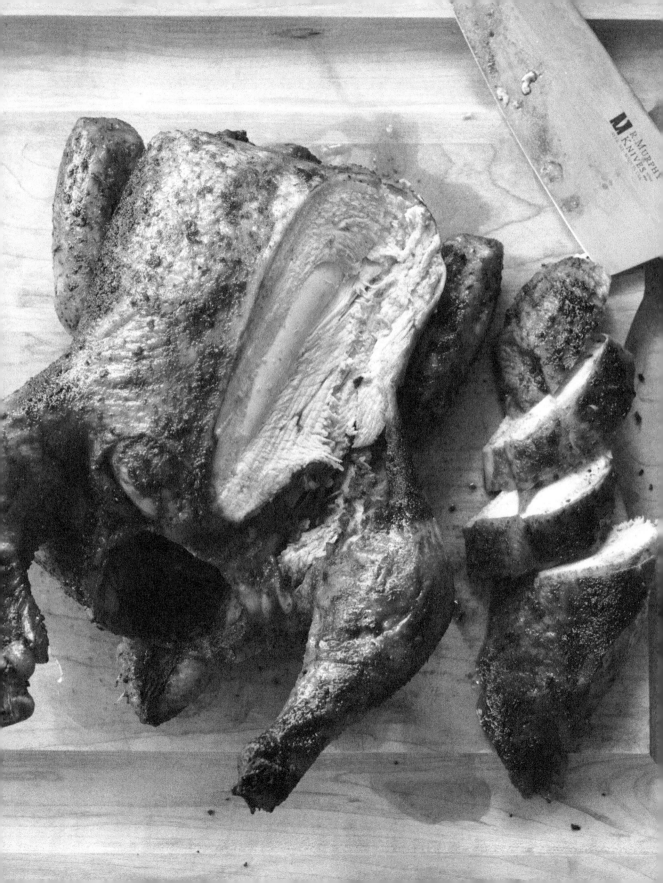

7

MEAT AND POULTRY

TURKEY PICCATA

ONE-POT Serve this turkey piccata with a side of cooked rice and some steamed veggies, and you've got a quick, easy, and healthy FODMAP-friendly meal. Because you pound the turkey thin, it cooks fast so you're ready to eat in no time. To pound the turkey, place it between two pieces of plastic wrap or parchment paper and pound it with a mallet or rolling pin—or anything else you have in your kitchen that will work well for this purpose (my mom always used a pot lid). *Serves 6*

PREP 10 minutes
COOK 15 minutes

1 (2-pound) turkey breast, cut into ½-inch-thick slices and pounded ⅛-inch thick

½ teaspoon sea salt

⅛ teaspoon freshly ground black pepper

½ cup King Arthur gluten-free flour

2 tablespoons extra-virgin olive oil

6 scallions (green part only), minced

1 cup dry white wine

Zest of 1 lemon

Juice of 1 lemon

2 tablespoons cold unsalted butter, cut into pieces

2 tablespoons chopped fresh parsley

1. Season the turkey breast slices with the sea salt and pepper, then coat with the flour, patting off any excess.

2. In a large skillet or sauté pan over medium-high heat, heat the olive oil until it shimmers.

3. Working in batches, brown the turkey slices in the hot oil for about 1 minute per side. Transfer to a plate tented with aluminum foil to keep them warm.

4. To the skillet, add the scallions, white wine, lemon zest, and lemon juice, using a spoon to scrape up any flavorful browned bits from the bottom of the skillet. Simmer for about 3 minutes, stirring occasionally, until the liquid is reduced by half.

5. One piece at a time, stir in the butter until incorporated.

6. Stir in the parsley. Spoon the sauce over the turkey.

for **PLAN A** Reduce the olive oil and unsalted butter to 1 tablespoon each. Replace the lemon juice with ¼ cup broth, but use the lemon zest. Eliminate the black pepper. Reduce the serving size by half or eat 1 full serving in 2 meals, 2 to 3 hours apart, to avoid overfilling your stomach.

for **PLAN D** Instead of coating the turkey with flour and sautéing it, cut the turkey into small pieces and simmer it in 2 cups broth for 15 to 20 minutes. Make the sauce as directed, starting at step 4.

PER SERVING Calories: 306; Total fat: 11g; Saturated fat: 4g; Carbohydrates: 16g; Fiber: 1g; Protein: 27g

GROUND TURKEY STIR-FRY

MAKE AHEAD | **ONE-POT** | **PORTABLE** You can cook a big batch of this dish and freeze it, or keep it in the refrigerator and reheat leftovers for meals on the go. It will keep for up to 3 days in the refrigerator or 12 months in the freezer. Store it in airtight single-serving containers so you always have just the right amount. *Serves 6*

PREP 10 minutes
COOK 15 minutes

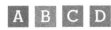

2 tablespoons Garlic Oil
(page 184)

1½ pounds ground turkey

1 tablespoon grated peeled
fresh ginger

6 scallions (green part
only), chopped

3 carrots, peeled and diced

3 cups fresh baby spinach

2 tablespoons gluten-free
soy sauce

Juice of 1 lime

2 tablespoons chopped
fresh cilantro

2 cups cooked brown
rice, warm

1. In a large skillet or sauté pan over medium-high, heat the garlic oil until it shimmers.

2. Add the turkey and ginger. Cook for about 5 minutes, stirring and crumbling with a spoon, until the turkey is browned.

3. Add the scallions and carrots. Cook for about 5 minutes more, stirring occasionally, until the veggies are soft.

4. Add the spinach. Cook, stirring, for 2 minutes.

5. Stir in the soy sauce and lime juice. Cook for 2 minutes.

6. Stir in the cilantro. Serve over the cooked rice.

for **PLAN A** Replace the garlic oil with 1 tablespoon extra-virgin olive oil. Reduce the serving size by half or eat 1 full serving in 2 meals, 2 to 3 hours apart, to avoid overfilling your stomach.

for **PLAN D** If garlic upsets your stomach, replace the garlic oil with extra-virgin olive oil. Precook the vegetables by simmering them for 5 to 10 minutes in 2 cups broth until they are soft. Drain the broth and add the cooked vegetables as indicated in the recipe. Replace the brown rice with white rice.

PER SERVING Calories: 398; Total fat: 17g; Saturated fat: 3g; Carbohydrates: 30g; Fiber: 2g; Protein: 35g

TURKEY MEATBALLS WITH GINGERED BOK CHOY

MAKE AHEAD As you bake the meatballs for this dinner, you can quickly cook the bok choy, which adds bright green color and a pop of flavor to this tasty dinner. You can also substitute any ground meat you like, such as chicken, pork, or beef, in place of the turkey. *Serves* 4

PREP 10 minutes
COOK 15 to 20 minutes

1 pound ground turkey breast

6 scallions (green part only), finely chopped

2 tablespoons chopped fresh cilantro

2 tablespoons grated peeled fresh ginger, divided

1 teaspoon mustard powder

1 teaspoon sea salt, divided

¼ teaspoon freshly ground black pepper, divided

2 pinches red pepper flakes, divided

1 large egg, beaten

1 slice Udi's gluten-free sandwich bread, processed into bread crumbs

2 tablespoons Garlic Oil (page 184)

1 head bok choy, chopped

1. Preheat the oven to 375°F.

2. Line a baking sheet with parchment paper.

3. In a large bowl, combine the turkey, scallions, cilantro, 1 tablespoon of ginger, mustard powder, ½ teaspoon of sea salt, ⅛ teaspoon of black pepper, 1 pinch of red pepper flakes, the egg, and bread crumbs. Mix until well combined. Roll the mixture into 1-inch balls and place on the prepared baking sheet. Bake for 15 to 20 minutes until cooked through.

4. Meanwhile, in a large skillet or sauté pan over medium-high heat, heat the garlic oil until it shimmers.

5. Add the bok choy, the remaining 1 tablespoon of ginger, ½ teaspoon of sea salt, ⅛ teaspoon of black pepper, and pinch of red pepper flakes. Cook for about 5 minutes, stirring occasionally, until the bok choy is soft.

for **PLAN A** Replace the garlic oil with 1 tablespoon extra-virgin olive oil. Eliminate the black pepper and red pepper flakes. Reduce the serving size by half or eat 1 full serving in 2 meals, 2 to 3 hours apart, to avoid overfilling your stomach.

for **PLAN C** Use whole-grain gluten-free bread to make the bread crumbs.

for **PLAN D** If garlic upsets your stomach, replace the garlic oil with extra-virgin olive oil. Cook the bok choy as directed. After 5 minutes, add ¼ cup broth and continue cooking until the liquid evaporates, to further soften the bok choy.

BIG 8 ALLERGENS Replace the egg with a flaxseed egg (see page 28).

PER SERVING Calories: 354; Total fat: 17g; Saturated fat: 4g; Carbohydrates: 11g; Fiber: 3g; Protein: 39g

ORANGE CHICKEN AND VEGGIE STIR-FRY

MAKE AHEAD | **ONE-POT** | **PORTABLE** Stir-frying is a great way to cook family meals, because recipes cook quickly and you can customize them with all kinds of ingredients to fit your own needs and your family's preferences. This version adds a tasty orange sauce to chicken and veggies. Serve it with steamed rice. *Serves 6*

PREP 10 minutes
COOK 15 minutes

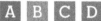

2 tablespoons Garlic Oil (page 184)

1 tablespoon grated peeled fresh ginger

1½ pounds boneless skinless chicken breast, cut into 1-inch pieces

2 red bell peppers, seeded and chopped

2 carrots, peeled and chopped

2 cups shredded green cabbage

2 tablespoons cornstarch

1 tablespoon gluten-free soy sauce

Juice of 1 orange

Pinch red pepper flakes

1. In a large skillet, sauté pan, or wok over medium-high heat, heat the garlic oil until it shimmers.

2. Add the ginger, chicken, red bell peppers, and carrots. Cook for 7 to 10 minutes, stirring occasionally, until the chicken and veggies are cooked.

3. Add the cabbage. Cook for 2 minutes more, stirring occasionally.

4. In a small bowl, whisk together the cornstarch, soy sauce, orange juice, and red pepper flakes. Add this slurry to the chicken and vegetables. Cook for 1 to 2 minutes more, stirring constantly, until the sauce thickens.

for **PLAN A** Replace the garlic oil with 1 tablespoon extra-virgin olive oil. Eliminate the red pepper flakes. Replace the orange juice with ½ cup broth and the zest of ½ orange. Reduce the serving size by half or eat 1 full serving in 2 meals, 2 to 3 hours apart, to avoid overfilling your stomach.

for **PLAN D** If garlic upsets your stomach, replace the garlic oil with extra-virgin olive oil. Eliminate the cabbage and red pepper flakes. Parcook the chicken, bell peppers, and carrots by simmering them in 2 cups broth for 15 minutes before adding to the stir-fry.

PER SERVING Calories: 301; Total fat: 11g; Saturated fat: 1g; Carbohydrates: 10g; Fiber: 2g; Protein: 34g

ARROZ CON POLLO

MAKE AHEAD | PORTABLE Arroz con pollo, which means chicken with rice in Spanish, is a traditional dish filled with Latin American flavors. This version is a quick stove-top sauté—it cooks fast but has lots of taste. Use purchased cooked rice or precooked rice, frozen and thawed, to save yourself time. *Serves 4*

PREP 10 minutes
COOK 15 minutes

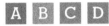

2 tablespoons Garlic Oil
(page 184)

1 pound boneless skinless
chicken breast, cut into
1-inch pieces

6 scallions (green part only),
finely chopped

2 green bell peppers, seeded
and chopped

1 (14-ounce) can
tomato sauce

½ cup Poultry Broth
(page 183)

Zest of 1 lime

Juice of 1 lime

1 teaspoon ground cumin

½ teaspoon chili powder

¼ cup chopped fresh cilantro

2 cups cooked brown rice

1 ounce Cheddar cheese,
grated (optional)

1. In a large skillet or sauté pan over medium-high heat, heat the garlic oil until it shimmers.

2. Add the chicken, scallions, and green bell peppers. Cook for 5 to 7 minutes, stirring occasionally, until the chicken and veggies are cooked.

3. Stir in the tomato sauce, broth, lime zest, lime juice, cumin, and chili powder. Cook for 5 minutes more, stirring occasionally.

4. Stir in the cilantro. Serve spooned over the rice and topped with Cheddar cheese (if using).

for **PLAN A** This dish is not GERD-friendly. But you can modify it to a more friendly state by replacing the tomato sauce with 3 cups broth and eliminate the lime juice. Then, at the end, stir in 2 tablespoons cornstarch whisked with 2 tablespoons water, to thicken the sauce. Eliminate the cheese. Reduce the serving size by half or eat 1 full serving in 2 meals, 2 to 3 hours apart, to avoid overfilling your stomach.

for **PLAN D** If garlic upsets your stomach, replace the garlic oil with extra-virgin olive oil. Eliminate the chili powder. Replace the brown rice with white rice. Increase the broth to 1 cup. Instead of performing step 2, simmer the chicken and vegetables in the broth, tomato sauce, and seasonings, covered, for 10 to 15 minutes, stirring occasionally, until the chicken and vegetables are very soft.

PER SERVING Calories: 534; Total fat: 20g; Saturated fat: 5g; Carbohydrates: 47g; Fiber: 5g; Protein: 41g

PORK TENDERLOIN WITH ASIAN SLAW

MAKE AHEAD The refreshing Asian slaw serves as the perfect counterpoint for the slightly sweet, earthy flavor of the pork in this recipe. You can cook the pork ahead and reheat it. If you make the slaw ahead, wait to add the vinaigrette until just before serving. *Serves 4*

PREP 10 minutes
COOK 15 minutes, plus 10 minutes to rest

 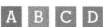

FOR THE PORK TENDERLOIN

2 tablespoons packed brown sugar

1 tablespoon grated peeled fresh ginger

Zest of 1 orange

1 teaspoon sea salt

1 teaspoon chili powder

½ teaspoon turmeric

⅛ teaspoon freshly ground black pepper

1 (1½-pound) pork tenderloin

1 tablespoon Garlic Oil (page 184)

FOR THE ASIAN SLAW

6 cups shredded cabbage

½ cup Asian Ginger Vinaigrette (page 186)

TO MAKE THE PORK TENDERLOIN

1. Preheat the oven to 400°F.

2. In a small bowl, whisk together the brown sugar, ginger, orange zest, sea salt, chili powder, turmeric, and pepper.

3. Brush the tenderloin with the garlic oil and then rub it with the spice mixture. Place it on a baking sheet and roast it for about 15 minutes. Turn halfway through cooking. Let it rest for 10 minutes before slicing.

TO MAKE THE ASIAN SLAW

In a large bowl, toss the cabbage with the vinaigrette and serve with the sliced pork.

for **PLAN A** Modify the Asian Ginger Vinaigrette as noted on page 186. Replace the chili powder with cumin and eliminate the black pepper. Don't rub the tenderloin with oil; add the rub directly to the tenderloin. Reduce the serving size by half or eat 1 full serving in 2 meals, 2 to 3 hours apart, to avoid over-filling your stomach.

for **PLAN D** Instead of making a slaw, sauté the cabbage in 2 tablespoons garlic oil for 4 minutes, stirring occasionally. Then squeeze in the juice of 1 orange and add ½ teaspoon grated peeled fresh ginger. Cook, covered, until the cabbage is soft. Instead of rubbing the tenderloin and roasting it, cut it into small pieces and simmer for 20 to 25 minutes, covered, in 4 cups broth, with the rub spices (minus the chili powder and garlic oil) added, until the meat is soft and well cooked.

PER SERVING Calories: 496; Total fat: 29g; Saturated fat: 5g; Carbohydrates: 12g; Fiber: 3g; Protein: 46g

PORK CHOPS WITH RHUBARB SAUCE

MAKE AHEAD Rhubarb sauce serves as a sweet grace note for the savory pork chops in this dish. You can make the rhubarb sauce ahead of time. It will keep refrigerated for 3 days in an airtight container, or you can freeze it for up to 1 year. Making a large batch ahead is a definite time-saver. *Serves 4*

PREP 15 minutes
COOK 15 minutes

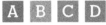

¼ cup water

⅓ cup sugar

2¼ cups chopped rhubarb

Zest of 1 lemon

Pinch ground nutmeg

¼ cup King Arthur gluten-free flour

1 teaspoon ground sage

1 teaspoon sea salt

⅛ teaspoon freshly ground black pepper

4 (4- to 6-ounce) thin-cut pork chops

2 tablespoons extra-virgin olive oil

1. In a medium pot over high heat, bring the water and sugar to a boil.

2. Stir in the rhubarb, lemon zest, and nutmeg. Reduce the heat to low and simmer for about 7 minutes, stirring occasionally, until the rhubarb is tender.

3. In a small shallow bowl, mix the flour, sage, sea salt, and pepper. Dip the pork chops in the flour mixture, patting off any excess.

4. In a large skillet or sauté pan over medium-high heat, heat the olive oil until it shimmers.

5. Add the pork chops and cook for 2 to 3 minutes per side until browned on both sides. Serve topped with the rhubarb sauce.

for **PLAN A** Reduce the olive oil to 1 tablespoon. Eliminate the black pepper. Reduce the serving size by half or eat 1 full serving in 2 meals, 2 to 3 hours apart, to avoid overfilling your stomach.

for **PLAN D** Replace the pork chops with pork tenderloin or pork shoulder cut into ½-inch pieces. Simmer the pork for about 15 minutes, covered, in 2 cups broth with the ground sage, sea salt, and pepper until cooked and soft.

PER SERVING Calories: 529; Total fat: 36g; Saturated fat: 12g; Carbohydrates: 25g; Fiber: 2g; Protein: 27g

HEARTY MEATLOAF

MAKE AHEAD | PORTABLE Serve this meatloaf with Loaded Smashed Potatoes (page 110) and a side of steamed veggies for a cozy family meal. Meatloaf is a classic family favorite, and this version is both flavorful and low-FODMAP. It's also easy to make, needing only a short amount of prep time. Most of the time is inactive while the meatloaf cooks in the oven. *Serves 6*

PREP 15 minutes
COOK 1 hour to 1 hour, 20 minutes

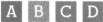

2 tablespoons Garlic Oil (page 184)

1 leek (green part only), finely chopped

4 slices Udi's gluten-free sandwich bread, processed into bread crumbs

1 cup unsweetened rice milk

1 pound ground beef

½ pound ground pork

2 large eggs, beaten

1 tablespoon Dijon mustard

1 tablespoon prepared horseradish

1 teaspoon dried thyme

1 teaspoon sea salt

¼ teaspoon freshly ground black pepper

1. Preheat the oven to 350°F.

2. Line a baking sheet with aluminum foil.

3. In a large skillet or sauté pan over medium-high heat, heat the garlic oil until it shimmers.

4. Add the leek and cook for 7 to 10 minutes, stirring frequently, until soft. Cool completely.

5. In a small bowl, mix the bread crumbs with the rice milk and set aside for 5 minutes.

6. In a large bowl, combine the beef, pork, eggs, Dijon mustard, horseradish, thyme, sea salt, pepper, leek, and bread crumb mixture. Mix until well combined.

7. Mold the meatloaf into a free-form oval-shaped loaf on the prepared baking sheet. Bake for 1 hour to 1 hour, 10 minutes until cooked through.

for **PLAN A** Replace the garlic oil with 1 tablespoon extra-virgin olive oil. Eliminate the black pepper. Use very lean ground beef and eliminate the ground pork. Reduce the serving size by half or eat 1 full serving in 2 meals, 2 to 3 hours apart, to avoid overfilling your stomach.

for **PLAN C** Make the bread crumbs with Udi's whole-grain gluten-free bread, or use cooked brown rice (1 cup).

for **PLAN D** If garlic upsets your stomach, replace the garlic oil with extra-virgin olive oil. Use lean ground beef, and replace the ground pork with ground beef. Eliminate the horseradish.

PER SERVING Calories: 426; Total fat: 16g; Saturated fat: 4g; Carbohydrates: 23g; Fiber: 1g; Protein: 45g

SPAGHETTI AND MEATBALLS

MAKE AHEAD | ONE-POT One of the issues with eating pasta on a low-FODMAP elimination diet is finding pasta that is low in FODMAPs, since most is made with wheat, and many alternative pastas use legume flour. While you can use corn pasta (read the labels), you can eliminate the worry altogether by using zucchini noodles. To make the noodles, use a spiralizer or julienne peeler. Or use a vegetable peeler to cut the zucchini into ribbons and then use a sharp knife to cut the ribbons into noodles. *Serves 6*

PREP 15 minutes
COOK 25 minutes

1 pound ground turkey

6 scallions (green part only), minced

2 slices Udi's gluten-free sandwich bread, processed into bread crumbs

1 large egg, beaten

1 tablespoon dried Italian seasoning

1 teaspoon sea salt, divided

⅛ teaspoon freshly ground black pepper

2 tablespoons Garlic Oil (page 184)

1 (14-ounce) can tomato sauce

1 (14-ounce) can crushed tomatoes, with juice

Pinch red pepper flakes

¼ cup chopped fresh basil

4 medium zucchini, spiralized

1. In a large bowl, mix the turkey, scallions, bread crumbs, egg, Italian seasoning, ½ teaspoon of sea salt, and the pepper. Roll the mixture into 1-inch balls and set them aside on a plate.

2. In a large pot over medium-high heat, heat the garlic oil until it shimmers.

3. Add the meatballs and cook for about 10 minutes, turning them as they brown.

4. Stir in the tomato sauce, crushed tomatoes and their juice, red pepper flakes, and the remaining ½ teaspoon of sea salt. Bring to a simmer. Cover, reduce the heat to low, and simmer for 10 minutes.

5. Add the zucchini noodles. Cook for 5 minutes more, or until the zucchini is al dente.

for **PLAN A** This recipe does not work for GERD because of the tomatoes, which are quite acidic. With modifications, you can enjoy the meatballs and the zucchini, however. Cook the meatballs in extra-virgin olive oil instead of garlic oil, and use lean ground beef only, not pork.

for **PLAN D** If garlic upsets your stomach, replace the garlic oil with extra-virgin olive oil. Eliminate the red pepper flakes. Peel the zucchini before spiralizing. Make the meatballs only ½ inch in size so they cook to a softer texture. Simmer the noodles for about 7 minutes to make them softer.

PER SERVING Calories: 395; Total fat: 9g; Saturated fat: 3g; Carbohydrates: 37g; Fiber: 9g; Protein: 43g

BEEF FAJITAS

Sizzling fajitas make dinnertime fun time. While onions don't fit in a low-FODMAP diet, bell peppers do, so you can still have a flavorful fajita without the FODMAPs that upset your stomach. *Serves 4*

PREP 15 minutes, plus 4 hours to marinate
COOK 15 minutes

6 scallions (green part only), chopped

1 jalapeño pepper, seeded and chopped

¼ cup fresh cilantro

Juice of 2 limes

4 tablespoons Garlic Oil (page 184), divided

½ teaspoon sea salt

1 (1-pound) flank steak

2 red bell peppers, seeded and sliced

2 green bell peppers, seeded and sliced

4 corn tortillas

1 avocado, pitted, peeled, and sliced

1. In a food processor or blender, combine the scallions, jalapeño, cilantro, lime juice, 3 tablespoons of garlic oil, and the sea salt. Process to a paste. Set aside 1 tablespoon of the paste. Transfer the rest to a large resealable bag.

2. Add the flank steak to the bag, turning to coat the steak with the paste. Refrigerate for 4 hours.

3. Wipe the paste from the steak. Heat a large skillet or sauté pan over medium-high heat and add the remaining 1 tablespoon of garlic oil to coat the skillet.

4. Add the steak to the hot skillet. Cook for about 5 minutes per side until it is medium-rare (145°F). Transfer to a cutting board and let it rest for 5 minutes.

5. Return the skillet to the heat and add the red bell peppers and the green bell peppers. Cook for about 5 minutes, stirring frequently, until soft.

6. Cut the steak against the grain into ½-inch-thick slices. Return to the skillet with the bell peppers.

7. Stir in the reserved paste, stir, and cook for 1 minute. Serve with the corn tortillas and sliced avocado.

for **PLAN A** This recipe is not GERD-friendly, so avoid it.

for **PLAN D** Eliminate the jalapeño and replace the garlic oil with extra-virgin olive oil. Wrap the meat in aluminum foil or an oven bag and roast it in a 375°F oven for about 30 minutes until very soft. Cut the meat against the grain into ¼-inch slices. Replace the green bell peppers with red bell peppers. Eliminate the corn tortillas and serve with the avocados and steamed white rice.

PER SERVING Calories: 536; Total fat: 34g; Saturated fat: 8g; Carbohydrates: 23g; Fiber: 8g; Protein: 35g

BISTRO BURGERS

PORTABLE What's special about these burgers? The amazing bistro sauce—which adds a sweet, savory flavor to the burger. The fish sauce also adds a unique savory quality, although you can eliminate it if you wish. *Serves 4*

PREP 15 minutes
COOK 15 minutes

1 pound ground turkey

½ teaspoon fish sauce

½ teaspoon sea salt

⅛ teaspoon freshly ground black pepper

1 teaspoon sugar

4 Udi's gluten-free hamburger buns

¼ cup Mayonnaise (page 178)

2 tablespoons packed brown sugar

1 tablespoon gluten-free soy sauce

1 tablespoon Worcestershire sauce

1 tablespoon chopped fresh chives

1. Preheat the oven to 450°F.

2. Place a metal rack on a baking sheet.

3. In a large bowl, mix the turkey, fish sauce, sea salt, pepper, and sugar. Form the mixture into 4 patties and place them on the rack.

4. Bake the burgers for about 15 minutes until they reach an internal temperature of 140°F (medium-rare) to 160°F (medium-well). Meanwhile, toast the buns if you wish.

5. In a small bowl, whisk the mayonnaise, brown sugar, soy sauce, Worcestershire sauce, and chives. Spread the sauce on the buns, and top with the burgers.

for **PLAN A** Eliminate the black pepper. Replace the mayonnaise with plain coconut yogurt or low-fat mayonnaise. Reduce the serving size by half or eat 1 full serving in 2 meals, 2 to 3 hours apart, to avoid overfilling your stomach.

for **PLAN C** Replace the buns with Udi's whole-grain gluten-free hamburger buns.

BIG-8 ALLERGENS If you are allergic to fish, eliminate the fish sauce.

PER SERVING Calories: 345; Total fat: 16g; Saturated fat: 6g; Carbohydrates: 11g; Fiber: 0g; Protein: 37g

BAKED MEDITERRANEAN TURKEY MEATBALLS WITH ROASTED RED PEPPER SAUCE

These turkey meatballs are loaded with savory Mediterranean flavors, while the red pepper sauce comes together quickly and adds a subtle sweetness to the finished dish. This recipe will fill your home with fragrant spices as it cooks. *Serves 4*

PREP 15 minutes
COOK 10 to 15 minutes

1 pound ground turkey

1 teaspoon ground cumin

1 teaspoon dried oregano

½ teaspoon sea salt

½ teaspoon ground coriander

½ teaspoon ground allspice

½ teaspoon ground ginger

⅛ teaspoon freshly ground black pepper

1 (28-ounce) can or jar roasted red peppers, drained

2 tablespoons Garlic Oil (page 184)

1. Preheat the oven to 400°F.

2. In a large bowl, mix the turkey, cumin, oregano, sea salt, coriander, allspice, ginger, and black pepper until well combined. Form the mixture into 1-inch balls and place them in a baking pan. Bake for 10 to 15 minutes until cooked through.

3. In a food processor or blender, combine the roasted red peppers and garlic oil. Process until smooth. Gently warm in a small pot over medium heat. Serve the meatballs topped with the red pepper sauce.

for **PLAN A** Eliminate the red pepper sauce, black pepper, and garlic oil. Reduce the serving size by half or eat 1 full serving in 2 meals, 2 to 3 hours apart, to avoid overfilling your stomach.

for **PLAN D** If garlic upsets your stomach, replace the garlic oil with extra-virgin olive oil.

PER SERVING Calories: 273; Total fat: 9g; Saturated fat: 3g; Carbohydrates: 14g; Fiber: 3g; Protein: 34g

ZUCCHINI LASAGNA

PORTABLE | MAKE AHEAD When that lasagna craving hits (you know what I mean!), don't fret about the pesky pasta. This recipe uses fresh zucchini in its place to keep your diet FODMAP-friendly. You can make this lasagna ahead of time and refrigerate it for up to 3 days before baking it. If you do so, let it sit on the counter for 30 minutes before you cook it. *Serves 6*

PREP 15 minutes
COOK 1 hour

2 (14-ounce) cans crushed tomatoes, in juice

2 tablespoons Garlic Oil (page 184)

1 tablespoon dried Italian seasoning

Pinch red pepper flakes

½ teaspoon sea salt

¼ teaspoon freshly ground black pepper

1 pound ground beef

4 large zucchini, cut into ribbons with a vegetable peeler

1 pound frozen spinach, thawed and squeezed of excess water

4 ounces Swiss cheese, grated

1. Preheat the oven to 350°F.

2. In a food processor or blender, combine the tomatoes and their juice, garlic oil, Italian seasoning, red pepper flakes, sea salt, and pepper. Process until smooth.

3. In a large skillet or sauté pan over medium-high heat, brown the ground beef for about 5 minutes, stirring and crumbling it with a spoon, until cooked.

4. In a 9-inch-square pan, spread one-third of the tomato sauce. Place one-third of the zucchini ribbons on top. Spread half of the ground beef over the zucchini, followed by half of the spinach, and one-third of the Swiss cheese.

5. Top with another third of the zucchini noodles, another third of the tomato sauce, the remaining half of the ground beef, the remaining half of the spinach, and another third of the cheese.

6. Finish with the remaining zucchini noodles, tomato sauce, and cheese. Cover with aluminum foil.

7. Bake for 45 minutes. Remove the foil and bake for 15 minutes more until the cheese is browned and bubbly.

for **PLAN A** This recipe is not GERD-friendly, so avoid it.

for **PLAN D** If garlic upsets your stomach, replace the garlic oil with extra-virgin olive oil. Leave the foil in place the whole time the casserole cooks. Peel the zucchini before cutting it into noodles and boil them in water for 3 minutes before adding to the recipe. Reduce the spinach to ½ pound.

PER SERVING Calories: 351; Total fat: 16g; Saturated fat: 6g; Carbohydrates: 19g; Fiber: 7g; Protein: 35g

COTTAGE PIE

PORTABLE Also called shepherd's pie, cottage pie comes from the UK. Traditionally, it's a combination of lamb, peas, and carrots topped with whipped potatoes. Here, we use ground lamb and eliminate high-FODMAP peas to make it FODMAP-friendly. *Serves 4*

PREP 15 minutes
COOK 50 minutes

1 pound potatoes, peeled and cut into 1-inch cubes

¼ cup unsweetened rice milk

2 tablespoons unsalted butter

1 teaspoon sea salt, divided

¼ teaspoon freshly ground black pepper, divided

1 ounce Cheddar cheese, grated

2 tablespoons Garlic Oil (page 184)

1 pound ground lamb

3 carrots, peeled and diced

1 leek (green part only), minced

1 fennel bulb, diced

1 teaspoon dried thyme

1. Preheat the oven to 400°F.

2. In a large pot of boiling water over high heat, boil the potatoes for 15 minutes until soft. Drain the potatoes and return them to the pot.

3. Add the rice milk, butter, ½ teaspoon of sea salt, and ⅛ teaspoon of pepper. Mash or whip until smooth.

4. Stir in the Cheddar cheese and set aside.

5. In a large skillet or sauté pan over medium-high heat, heat the garlic oil until it shimmers.

6. Add the lamb and cook for about 5 minutes, stirring and crumbling the meat with a spoon, until browned.

7. Stir in the carrots, leek, fennel, and thyme. Cook for 5 minutes more, stirring occasionally. Spoon the mixture into a 9-inch-square baking pan. Spread the potatoes across the top.

8. Bake for 25 minutes until the potatoes are browned.

for **PLAN A** Eliminate the black pepper, butter, and Cheddar cheese, and replace the garlic oil with 1 tablespoon extra-virgin olive oil. Reduce the serving size by half or eat 1 full serving in 2 meals, 2 to 3 hours apart, to avoid overfilling your stomach.

for **PLAN D** Eliminate the leeks and fennel. Increase the carrots to 5 and precook them by boiling for 10 minutes in broth. Drain before adding to the lamb. Omit the Cheddar cheese. If garlic upsets your stomach, replace the garlic oil with extra-virgin olive oil.

BIG-8 ALLERGENS If you're allergic to dairy, replace the butter with 2 tablespoons garlic oil and eliminate the Cheddar cheese.

PER SERVING Calories: 481; Total fat: 24g; Saturated fat: 9g; Carbohydrates: 30g; Fiber: 6g; Protein: 37g

ROASTED CHICKEN WITH ROOT VEGETABLES

ONE-POT What smells so good? This simple Sunday-style dinner, which takes only a few moments to prepare but results in a delicious meal that tastes like you fussed all day. You can use a roasting pan, or, if you have one, a large enameled cast iron Dutch oven to prepare this meal. *Serves 4*

PREP 15 minutes
COOK 1 hour, 15 minutes

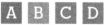

1 (4-pound) roasting chicken

Sea salt

Freshly ground black pepper

1 fresh rosemary sprig

1 fresh thyme sprig

3 scallions (green part only)

1 lemon, halved

3 carrots, peeled and chopped into 1-inch pieces

4 small new red potatoes, chopped into 1-inch pieces

1. Preheat the oven to 350°F.

2. Season the chicken with sea salt and pepper. Stuff the rosemary, thyme, scallions, and lemon halves into the cavity.

3. In a roasting pan, place the carrots and potatoes in an even layer. Top with a roasting rack and place the chicken on the rack.

4. Bake for about 1 hour, 15 minutes until the juices run clear when you pierce the thigh with the tip of a sharp knife. Let it rest for 10 minutes before carving and serving.

for **PLAN A** Eliminate the black pepper. Remove the chicken skin before serving. Eat the white meat only. Reduce the serving size by half or eat 1 full serving in 2 meals, 2 to 3 hours apart, to avoid overfilling your stomach.

for **PLAN D** Remove the chicken skin before serving. Eat the white meat only.

PER SERVING Calories: 481; Total fat: 24g; Saturated fat: 9g; Carbohydrates: 30g; Fiber: 6g; Protein: 37g

PAN-SEARED CHICKEN BREAST WITH AVOCADO-TOMATO SALSA

Dress your chicken to impress. This fresh-tasting salsa pairs perfectly with protein-rich chicken, and dinner is on the table in less than 30 minutes. You need an ovenproof skillet for this. A stainless steel or cast iron skillet is a good choice. *Serves 4*

PREP 5 minutes
COOK 25 minutes

FOR THE CHICKEN

2 tablespoons extra-virgin olive oil

4 (4-ounce) boneless skinless chicken breasts

½ teaspoon sea salt

⅛ teaspoon freshly ground black pepper

FOR THE SALSA

1 medium tomato, finely chopped

½ avocado, peeled, pitted, and finely chopped

1 teaspoon Garlic Oil (page 184)

1 tablespoon freshly squeezed lime juice

TO MAKE THE CHICKEN

1. Preheat the oven to 400°F.

2. In an ovenproof skillet over medium-high heat, heat the olive oil until it shimmers.

3. Season the chicken with sea salt and pepper and add it to the skillet. Cook the chicken for about 5 minutes without moving it. Flip and cook on the other side for 5 minutes more.

4. Transfer the skillet to the oven and cook for 10 to 15 minutes more until the juices run clear when you pierce a piece with the tip of a sharp knife.

TO MAKE THE SALSA

In a small bowl, stir together the tomato, avocado, garlic oil, and lime juice. Serve with the chicken.

for **PLAN A** This recipe is not GERD-friendly. While the chicken is, the salsa can trigger acid reflux.

for **PLAN D** You may want to alter the texture of this dish by cutting the chicken into 1-inch cubes and boiling it for about 15 minutes in 2 cups broth until done.

PER SERVING Calories: 342; Total fat: 22g; Saturated fat: 5g; Carbohydrates: 3g; Fiber: 2g; Protein: 34g

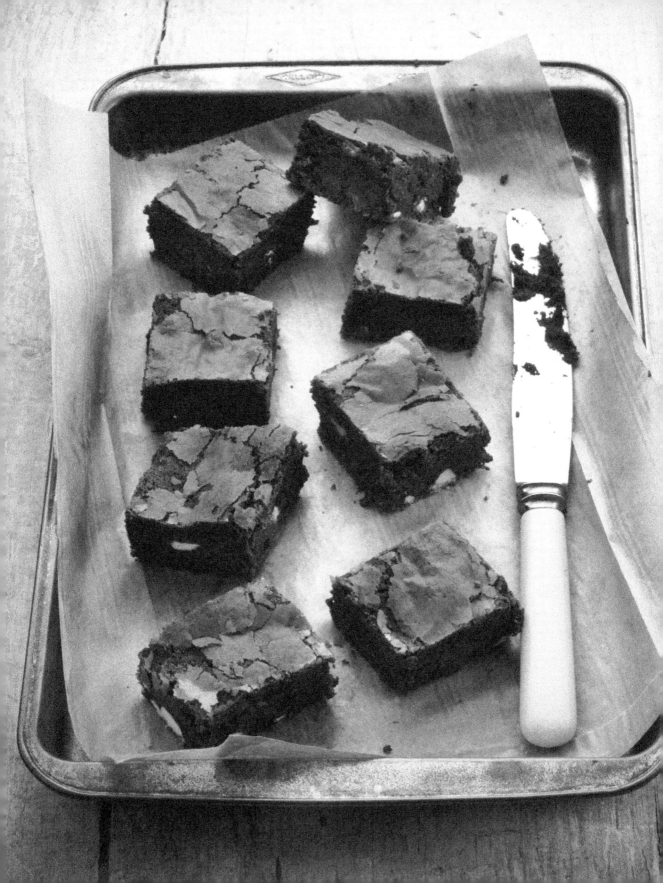

8

DESSERTS

COCONUT CUSTARD WITH BERRY SAUCE

MAKE AHEAD | **ONE-POT** | **PORTABLE** | **VEGAN** Coconut milk serves as the base for this flavorful, creamy pudding that will leave you wanting more. It's made just like a traditional pudding, thickened with cornstarch. The berry sauce adds rich sweetness, so this is a recipe your family will adore as a simple dessert or for a special occasion. *Serves 4*

PREP 5 minutes
COOK 10 minutes

2 cups canned full-fat coconut milk

¾ cup sugar, divided

Pinch sea salt

3 tablespoons cornstarch

3 tablespoons water

Juice of 1 orange

½ cup fresh blueberries

½ cup fresh raspberries

1. In a medium pot over medium-high heat, bring the coconut milk, ½ cup of sugar, and the sea salt to a boil while stirring.

2. In a small bowl, whisk together the cornstarch and water thoroughly. In a thin stream, slowly add this slurry to the boiling pudding, whisking constantly. Continue cooking, whisking constantly, for 1 to 2 minutes more until the pudding thickens. Spoon into 4 dessert dishes and refrigerate to cool.

3. In a medium pot over medium-high heat, heat the remaining ¼ cup of sugar, the orange juice, blueberries, and raspberries, stirring frequently. Reduce the heat and simmer for about 4 minutes, stirring occasionally until the berries thicken and are saucy.

4. Serve the chilled pudding with either warm or chilled berry sauce spooned over the top.

for **PLAN A** Use canned light coconut milk and include ½ teaspoon coconut extract. Eliminate the orange juice and replace it with ¼ cup water. Reduce the serving size by half or eat 1 full serving in 2 meals, 2 to 3 hours apart, to avoid overfilling your stomach.

PER SERVING Calories: 465; Total fat: 29g; Saturated fat: 25g; Carbohydrates: 56g; Fiber: 4g; Protein: 3g

CHOCOLATE PUDDING

PORTABLE | MAKE AHEAD | VEGAN Chocolate lovers rejoice! This rich chocolate pudding is a delicious part of a FODMAP-friendly diet, and you won't even notice it doesn't contain any dairy. You'll know the pudding is perfectly thick enough when it coats the back of a spoon and you can run your finger through the pudding on the spoon, leaving a trail. *Serves 4*

PREP 5 minutes
COOK 10 minutes

2¾ cups unsweetened rice milk

¼ cup unsweetened cocoa powder

½ cup sugar

¼ cup cornstarch

Pinch sea salt

1 teaspoon vanilla extract

1. In a medium pot, whisk the rice milk, cocoa powder, sugar, cornstarch, and sea salt.

2. Turn the heat to medium under the pot. Bring the mixture to a boil, stirring constantly. Continue to boil for 1 to 2 minutes more, stirring constantly, until the pudding thickens and coats the back of a spoon. Remove the pot from the heat and stir in the vanilla.

3. Chill before serving.

for **PLAN A** Chocolate can trigger GERD, so avoid this recipe.

PER SERVING Calories: 222; Total fat: 2g; Saturated fat: <1g; Carbohydrates: 52g; Fiber: 2g; Protein: 1g

PEANUT BUTTER COOKIES WITH DARK CHOCOLATE CHIPS

MAKE AHEAD | PORTABLE | VEGETARIAN If you're like me and you like (love!?) a good chocolate chip cookie, then you're in luck. These cookies are made without any flour, so they're low in FODMAPs. Be sure to use dark chocolate chips and double check that the ingredients don't include high fructose corn syrup, which may aggravate your condition. Choose unsweetened peanut butter, as well. *Makes 18 cookies*

PREP 5 minutes
COOK 10 minutes

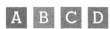

1 cup creamy peanut butter
½ cup granulated sugar
½ cup packed brown sugar
1 large egg, beaten
1 teaspoon vanilla extract
Pinch sea salt
1 cup dark chocolate chips

1. Preheat the oven to 350°F.

2. Line a baking sheet with parchment paper.

3. In a medium bowl, mix the peanut butter, granulated sugar, brown sugar, egg, vanilla, and sea salt until well combined.

4. Stir in the chocolate chips. Drop the batter by tablespoonfuls onto the prepared baking sheet, spaced about ½ inch apart. You should have 18 cookies.

5. Bake for about 10 minutes until golden.

for **PLAN A** Eliminate the chocolate chips.

BIG 8 ALLERGENS If you're allergic to peanut butter, avoid this recipe since there isn't a good substitute for peanut butter.

PER SERVING (1 cookie) Calories: 156; Total fat: 9g; Saturated fat: <3g; Carbohydrates: 17g; Fiber: <1g; Protein: 4g

LEMON-LIME GRANITA

MAKE AHEAD | **VEGAN** If they are in season, Meyer lemons are delicious in this refreshing granita because they have a sweet, ultra-lemony flavor. This refreshing dessert doesn't take much effort, and it's showy and flavorful, so it's perfect for summer entertaining—or for just entertaining your taste buds. *Serves 4*

PREP 10 minutes
COOK 5 minutes, plus 2 hours or more to steep and freeze

1 cup water
1 cup sugar
Zest of 2 large lemons
Juice of 2 large lemons
Zest of 1 lime
Juice of 1 lime

1. In a large pot over high heat, heat the water, sugar, lemon zest, lemon juice, lime zest, and lime juice for about 5 minutes, stirring, until the sugar dissolves. Remove from the heat and let steep for 15 minutes.

2. Strain the mixture through a fine-mesh sieve into a 9-by-5-inch loaf pan. Freeze, uncovered, for 1 hour.

3. Scrape with a fork to break up the ice crystals. Return to the freezer for 1 hour more. Scrape with a fork again. Continue this cycle until all the liquid is frozen and snowy.

for **PLAN A** This dessert is not GERD-friendly, so avoid it.

PER SERVING Calories: 195; Total fat: <1g; Saturated fat: 0g; Carbohydrates: 51g; Fiber: 0g; Protein: <1g

RASPBERRY GRANITA

MAKE AHEAD | **VEGAN** This raspberry granita tastes like fresh berry sorbet, both sweet and acidic at the same time. It's a delicious, refreshing ice that makes the perfect light cap to your low-FODMAP meal. *Serves 4*

PREP 10 minutes
COOK 5 minutes, plus
2 hours or more to steep
and freeze

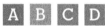

1 cup water
1 cup sugar
1 pint fresh raspberries
Zest of 1 orange

1. In a large pot over medium-high heat, combine the water, sugar, raspberries, and orange zest. Heat for about 5 minutes, stirring and mashing the raspberries with a spoon, until the sugar is dissolved and the raspberries are mushy.

2. Strain the mixture through a fine-mesh sieve into a 9-by-5-inch loaf pan. Discard the solids. Freeze, uncovered, for 1 hour. Scrape with a fork to break up the ice crystals. Return to the freezer for 1 hour more. Scrape with a fork again. Continue this cycle until all the liquid is frozen and snowy.

for **PLAN A** Reduce the serving size by half or eat 1 full serving in 2 meals, 2 to 3 hours apart, to avoid overfilling your stomach.

PER SERVING Calories: 228; Total fat: <1g; Saturated fat: 0g; Carbohydrates: 59g; Fiber: 5g; Protein: <1g

BERRIES AND CREAM

MAKE AHEAD | PORTABLE | VEGAN So simple, yet so delicious, you'll love this quick dessert. The trick with the cream is to have the coconut cream very chilled. You can get the coconut cream in one of two ways. Some stores sell canned coconut cream. If you can't find it, chill a can of full-fat coconut milk in the refrigerator overnight. The cream will separate from the liquid and rise to the top. Open the can and spoon the cream into a bowl and discard the watery liquid. *Serves 4*

PREP 10 minutes
COOK 0 minutes

1 cup canned coconut cream

1 tablespoon pure
maple syrup

½ teaspoon vanilla extract

1 cup fresh raspberries

1 cup fresh blueberries

1 cup fresh strawberries,
hulled and sliced

1. In a large bowl, whisk the coconut cream, maple syrup, and vanilla until well mixed.

2. Add the raspberries, blueberries, and strawberries and toss with the flavored cream. Serve chilled.

for **PLAN A** Cut the amount of coconut cream by half and use alcohol-free vanilla extract. Reduce the serving size by half or eat 1 full serving in 2 meals, 2 to 3 hours apart, to avoid overfilling your stomach.

for **PLAN D** Cook the berries in ¼ cup water over medium-high heat for about 5 minutes until they make a sauce. Strain the mixture through a fine-mesh sieve and discard the solids. Whisk the sauce into the coconut cream.

PER SERVING Calories: 201; Total fat: 15g; Saturated fat: 13g; Carbohydrates: 18g; Fiber: 5g; Protein: 2g

YOGURT AND BERRY PARFAITS

MAKE AHEAD | **PORTABLE** | **VEGETARIAN** Who says you can't eat dessert first? This delightful dessert also makes a delicious breakfast. While it doesn't require cooking, if you have IBD/IBS-D you may wish to cook, cool, and strain the berries to create a softer texture that has less fiber and is easier on your stomach. *Serves 4*

PREP 10 minutes
COOK 0 minutes

2 cups plain coconut yogurt, or lactose-free plain yogurt

2 tablespoons pure maple syrup

1 teaspoon orange zest

½ teaspoon vanilla extract

Pinch ground nutmeg

½ cup fresh raspberries

½ cup fresh blueberries

1. In a medium bowl, whisk together the yogurt, maple syrup, orange zest, vanilla, and nutmeg.

2. In 4 parfait cups, layer the raspberries and blueberries with the yogurt mixture.

for **PLAN A** Choose fat-free or low-fat yogurt and use alcohol-free vanilla extract. Reduce the serving size by half or eat 1 full serving in 2 meals, 2 to 3 hours apart, to avoid overfilling your stomach.

for **PLAN C** Add 2 tablespoons chopped walnuts or pecans to the parfait layers, to add fiber.

for **PLAN D** Cook the berries in ¼ cup water over medium-high heat for about 5 minutes until they make a sauce. Strain the mixture through a fine-mesh sieve and discard the solids. Layer the sauce with the yogurt.

PER SERVING Calories: 134; Total fat: 2g; Saturated fat: 1g; Carbohydrates: 20g; Fiber: 2g; Protein: 7g

FROZEN STRAWBERRY COCONUT BARS

MAKE AHEAD | PORTABLE | VEGAN If you don't have ice pop freezer containers, use paper cups. To do this, pour the mixture into the paper cups and place aluminum foil over the top. Insert ice pop sticks through the foil and freeze. Peel away the cups to serve. *Serves 6*

PREP 10 minutes
COOK 5 minutes, plus 3 to 4 hours to freeze

1 cup water

1 cup sugar

1 pint fresh strawberries, hulled and sliced

1 cup canned full-fat coconut milk

1. In a large saucepan over medium-high heat, heat the water, sugar, and strawberries, stirring frequently and mashing the strawberries with a spoon as you cook them. Simmer for 5 minutes, stirring frequently. Strain the mixture into a large bowl, discarding the solids.

2. Stir in the coconut milk.

3. Freeze in ice pop molds for 3 to 4 hours until frozen.

for **PLAN A** Use canned light coconut milk. Reduce the serving size by half or eat 1 full serving in 2 meals, 2 to 3 hours apart, to avoid overfilling your stomach.

for **PLAN C** Don't strain the strawberries. Instead, use a potato masher to make sure they are well incorporated into the syrup before adding the coconut milk. This adds fiber.

PER SERVING Calories: 236; Total fat: 10g; Saturated fat: 9g; Carbohydrates: 40g; Fiber: 2g; Protein: 1g

LEMON BARS

MAKE AHEAD | PORTABLE | VEGETARIAN Lemon bars are a glorious dessert, with a sweet and sour lemon filling and a tasty shortbread crust. This version has all the flavors you crave in this classic dessert, without the FODMAPs. *Makes 24 bars*

PREP 10 minutes
COOK 40 minutes, plus 1 hour to cool and chill

FOR THE CRUST

1¾ cups King Arthur gluten-free flour

⅔ cup powdered sugar

¼ cup cornstarch

½ teaspoon sea salt

½ cup (1 stick) very cold unsalted butter, cut into pieces, plus more for the pan

4 tablespoons very cold coconut oil, cut into pieces

FOR THE FILLING

4 large eggs

1⅓ cups sugar

3 tablespoons King Arthur gluten-free flour

Zest of 2 lemons

⅔ cup freshly squeezed lemon juice

⅓ cup unsweetened rice milk

Pinch sea salt

TO MAKE THE CRUST

1. Preheat the oven to 350°F. Coat a 9-by-13-inch baking dish with butter.

2. In a blender, combine the flour, powdered sugar, cornstarch, and sea salt and pulse 10 times, in 1-second bursts.

3. Add the butter and coconut oil. Pulse 4 to 5 times more, in 1-second bursts, until the mixture resembles sand. (Alternatively, use a pastry blender or two knives to cut the butter and coconut oil into the mixture until it resembles sand.) Transfer the mixture to the prepared pan, and press the crust into the bottom and slightly up the sides of the pan.

4. Bake for 15 to 20 minutes until just brown.

TO MAKE THE FILLING

1. While the crust bakes, in a medium bowl whisk the eggs, sugar, and flour. Stir in the lemon zest, rice milk, lemon juice, and sea salt. Pour the mixture into the warm crust.

2. Bake for about 20 minutes until the filling is set. Cool on a wire rack for 30 minutes. Refrigerate before cutting into bars and serving.

for **PLAN A** This is not GERD-friendly, so avoid it.

for **PLAN D** Skip the crust and bake squares of the filling.

BIG 8 ALLERGENS If you're allergic to dairy, eliminate the butter and increase the coconut oil by ½ cup.

PER SERVING Calories: 163; Total fat: 7g; Saturated fat: 5g; Carbohydrates: 24g; Fiber: 0g; Protein: 2g

CHOCOLATE-DIPPED STRAWBERRIES

MAKE AHEAD | **PORTABLE** | **VEGAN** Coconut oil helps the chocolate coating in this dessert harden to a lovely crunch. For GERD, try white chocolate in place of the dark chocolate— that way, you won't have to skip this yummy treat. Aside from strawberries, get creative and dip other fruits, such as citrus or melon wedges, for flavorful variations. *Serves 4*

PREP 10 minutes
COOK 5 minutes, plus
10 minutes to chill

4 ounces sweetened dark chocolate, cut into pieces

2 tablespoons coconut oil

12 large fresh strawberries, stems on

1. Line a baking sheet with parchment paper.

2. In a heavy medium saucepan over medium-high heat, melt the chocolate and coconut oil for about 5 minutes, stirring constantly, until melted. Remove from the heat.

3. Holding the stem end of the strawberries, dip them into the chocolate, leaving the stem end free of chocolate. Place them on the prepared pan to cool. To help the chocolate coating harden, put the pan in the refrigerator for 10 minutes.

for **PLAN A** Replace the dark chocolate with white chocolate. Reduce the serving size to 1 strawberry to avoid overfilling your stomach.

for **PLAN D** Try bananas instead of strawberries, as they have a softer texture.

PER SERVING (3 dipped strawberries) Calories: 228; Total fat: 15g; Saturated fat: 12g; Carbohydrates: 21g; Fiber: 2g; Protein: 3g

CHOCOLATE PEANUT BUTTER FUDGE PIE

MAKE AHEAD | **PORTABLE** | **VEGAN** Yes, you can have your pie and eat it, too. This simple pie is truly delicious—with a rich chocolate and peanut butter filling and a pecan–cocoa crust. It's bound to become a family favorite and nobody will suspect it's a special recipe that's low in FODMAPs. Choose sugar-free peanut butter. *Serves 8*

PREP 10 minutes
COOK 15 minutes, plus
1 hour to chill

FOR THE CRUST

1½ cups pecans,
finely chopped

¾ cup sugar

¼ cup unsweetened
cocoa powder

¼ cup coconut oil, melted,
plus more for the pan

FOR THE FILLING

¼ cup creamy peanut butter

4 ounces unsweetened
chocolate

2 cups canned
coconut cream

1 teaspoon vanilla extract

20 drops liquid stevia, or
as needed

TO MAKE THE CRUST

1. Preheat the oven to 350°F.

2. Coat a pie pan with coconut oil.

3. In a blender or food processor, combine the pecans, sugar, and cocoa powder. Pulse 10 to 20 times in 1-second bursts until the mixture is finely ground.

4. Add the coconut oil. Pulse 5 times more, in 1-second bursts. Press the crust into the prepared pan.

5. Bake for about 15 minutes until the crust is fragrant.

TO MAKE THE FILLING

1. In a medium saucepan over medium heat, melt the peanut butter and chocolate, stirring constantly. Remove from the heat and set aside.

2. In a large bowl, whisk the coconut cream, vanilla, and stevia until mixed.

3. Whisk in the chocolate and peanut butter mixture until well combined. Pour the filling into the crust and use a rubber spatula to spread it evenly. Refrigerate for 1 hour before slicing and serving.

for **PLAN A** This recipe is not GERD-friendly, so avoid it.

for **PLAN D** Skip the crust and pour the fudge mixture into a parchment-lined 8-inch-square pan. Refrigerate until firm and cut into 1-inch pieces of fudge.

BIG 8 ALLERGENS If you're allergic to tree nuts, replace the pecans with peanuts. If you are allergic to peanuts, there is no low-FODMAP substitution you can make here, so avoid this recipe.

PER SERVING Calories: 492; Total fat: 43g; Saturated fat: 25g; Carbohydrates: 31g; Fiber: 7g; Protein: 7g

RASPBERRY GELATIN

MAKE AHEAD | PORTABLE Gelatin is especially healing for damaged GI tracts, so this sweet dessert may also help heal what ails you. Use plain gelatin to mix with the raspberry sauce here—no need to buy boxes of Jell-O, which have all kinds of ingredients you don't want. *Serves 4*

PREP 10 minutes
COOK 5 minutes, plus 2 hours to cool

1½ cups water, at room temperature, divided

2 tablespoons gelatin

1 cup sugar

1 pint fresh raspberries

1. Line a 9-by-5-inch loaf pan with parchment paper and set aside.

2. In a small bowl, mix together ½ cup of water and the gelatin. Set aside.

3. In a medium saucepan over high heat, combine the remaining 1 cup of water, the sugar, and raspberries. Bring to a boil and cook for 5 minutes, stirring occasionally, until the sugar dissolves.

4. Strain the hot mixture into a large bowl, discarding the solids. Stir in the gelatin mixture until smooth.

5. Pour the mixture into the prepared loaf pan and refrigerate for 2 hours. To serve, lift the parchment paper–wrapped gelatin to a cutting board. Cut into squares.

for **PLAN A** Reduce the serving size by half or eat 1 full serving in 2 meals, 2 to 3 hours apart, to avoid overfilling your stomach.

for **PLAN C** Stir an additional ½ cup raspberries into the gelatin before refrigerating, to add fiber.

PER SERVING Calories: 181; Total fat: <1g; Saturated fat: 0g; Carbohydrates: 34g; Fiber: 5g; Protein: 13g

BANANA PUDDING

MAKE AHEAD | PORTABLE | VEGETARIAN Did you (or your mom) ever make the banana pudding recipe on the box of vanilla wafers—you know, that vanilla pudding, vanilla wafer, and banana dessert? This is like that, minus the cookies. This flavorful vanilla pudding is served with sliced bananas instead. *Serves 4*

PREP 10 minutes
COOK 8 minutes, plus 1 hour to chill

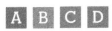

⅓ cup sugar

2 tablespoons cornstarch

Pinch sea salt

2¼ cups unsweetened rice milk, divided

3 large egg yolks, beaten

2 teaspoons vanilla extract

2 bananas, sliced, divided

1. In a medium saucepan, whisk the sugar, cornstarch, and sea salt.

2. In a thin stream while whisking constantly, pour in ¼ cup of rice milk.

3. Whisk in the egg yolks.

4. Whisk in the remaining 2 cups of rice milk until smooth.

5. Turn the heat to medium under the pan. Cook the pudding for about 5 minutes, stirring constantly, until it starts to thicken. Reduce the heat to low. Continue cooking for 3 minutes more, stirring constantly.

6. Remove from the heat and stir in the vanilla. Refrigerate for 1 hour before serving.

7. Using half of the banana slices, cover the bottoms of 4 ramekins. Spoon the pudding over the top and arrange the remaining banana slices on top of the pudding.

for **PLAN A** Reduce the serving size by half or eat 1 full serving in 2 meals, 2 to 3 hours apart, to avoid overfilling your stomach.

PER SERVING Calories: 244; Total fat: 5; Saturated fat: 1g; Carbohydrates: 48g; Fiber: 2g; Protein: 3g

LACTOSE-FREE ICE CREAM WITH SPICED BERRY SYRUP

MAKE AHEAD | **PORTABLE** | **VEGETARIAN** If you can't find ice cream that works with your diet, consider replacing it with plain Greek yogurt. While it isn't frozen, it's still delicious with the berry syrup and is a safe choice when you're minimizing FODMAPs. *Serves 4*

PREP 10 minutes
COOK 5 minutes, plus
10 minutes to steep

   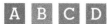

½ cup water

½ cup sugar

1 pint fresh raspberries

1 cinnamon stick

¼ teaspoon ground ginger

Pinch ground nutmeg

4 scoops lactose-free vanilla ice cream

1. In a medium saucepan over medium-high heat, heat the water, sugar, raspberries, cinnamon stick, ginger, and nutmeg, stirring occasionally and mashing the raspberries with a spoon.

2. Bring the mixture to a boil and cook for 5 minutes, stirring occasionally. Remove from the heat and let steep for 10 minutes. Strain the mixture through a fine-mesh sieve into a bowl, pressing on the berry solids to extract as much liquid as possible. Discard the solids.

3. Serve the warm berry syrup over the ice cream.

for **PLAN A** Reduce the serving size by half or eat 1 full serving in 2 meals, 2 to 3 hours apart, to avoid overfilling your stomach.

for **PLAN C** For additional fiber, use 2 tablespoons chopped pecans to sprinkle on top of the desserts.

BIG 8 ALLERGENS For dairy allergies, choose a nondairy ice cream.

PER SERVING Calories: 280; Total fat: 9g; Saturated fat: 5g; Carbohydrates: 51g; Fiber: 5g; Protein: 4g

BROWNIES

MAKE-AHEAD | ONE-POT | PORTABLE | VEGETARIAN There is no need to give up chewy, gooey brownies, even when on the strictest low-FODMAP elimination diet (unless you have GERD, because chocolate can trigger acid reflux). This recipe uses a wheat-free flour to keep FODMAPs low, while keeping overall brownie satisfaction high. *Makes 12 brownies*

PREP 15 minutes
COOK 35 to 40 minutes

1¼ cups sugar

6 tablespoons canola oil

¼ cup (½ stick) unsalted butter

⅔ cup unsweetened cocoa powder

½ teaspoon sea salt

1 teaspoon vanilla extract

2 large eggs

6 tablespoons King Arthur gluten-free flour

1. Preheat the oven to 350°F.

2. Line an 8-inch-square baking pan with parchment paper.

3. In a large saucepan over medium-high heat, combine the sugar, canola oil, butter, and cocoa powder. Cook for about 5 minutes, stirring frequently, until the butter is melted and the sugar has mostly dissolved.

4. Stir in the sea salt and vanilla, and remove from the heat.

5. One at a time, add the eggs, stirring to combine after each addition.

6. Stir in the flour until just mixed. Pour the batter into the prepared pan.

7. Bake for 30 to 35 minutes until a toothpick inserted into the center comes out clean.

for **PLAN A** This recipe is not GERD-friendly, so avoid it.

for **PLAN D** This recipe may be too rich for IBD/IBS-D, so proceed with caution.

PER SERVING Calories: 212; Total fat: 12g; Saturated fat: 4g; Carbohydrates: 27g; Fiber: 2g; Protein: 2g

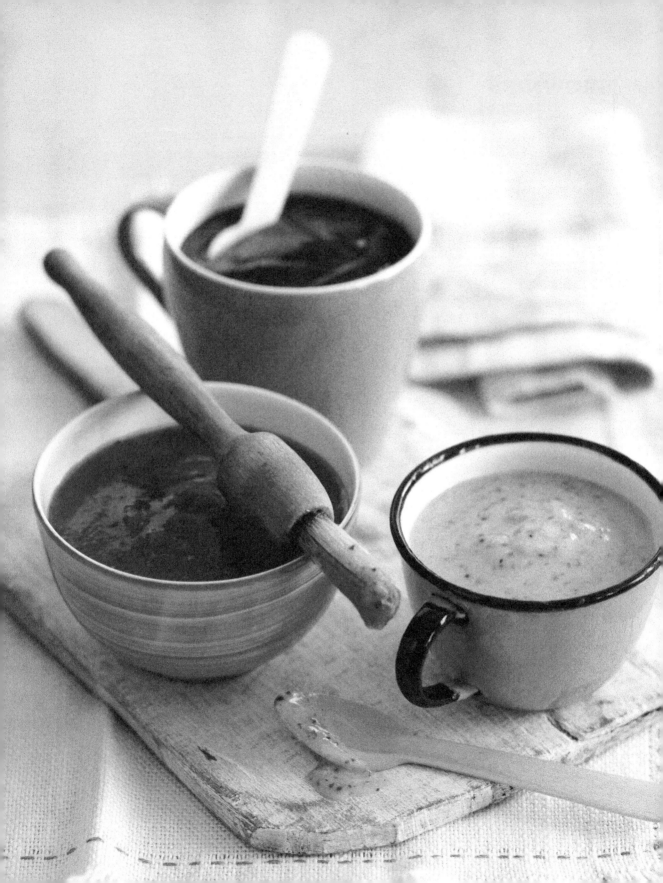

9

CONDIMENTS, SAUCES, AND DRESSINGS

MAYONNAISE

MAKE AHEAD | **ONE-POT** | **PORTABLE** | **VEGETARIAN** If you read the ingredients on a mayonnaise container, you may notice that most contain high fructose corn syrup, which is not FODMAP-friendly. Making your own mayonnaise is easy and quick, and it's completely FODMAP-friendly. *Makes ¾ cup*

PREP 5 minutes
COOK 0 minutes

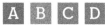

1 large pasteurized egg yolk

2 teaspoons white vinegar

½ teaspoon Dijon mustard

Pinch sea salt

¾ cup canola oil

1. In a blender or food processor, mix the egg yolk, white vinegar, Dijon mustard, and sea salt until well combined.

2. With the blender or food processor running, add the canola oil a drop at a time until you've incorporated about 10 drops. Then, slowly add the remaining oil in a very thin stream, processing constantly until all the oil is added and the dressing is emulsified. Refrigerate for up to 5 days.

for **PLAN A** Even though this recipe contains vinegar, it is such a small amount that it should not trigger GERD. But limit the mayo use to 1-tablespoon servings, because it is quite high in fat.

PER SERVING (1 tablespoon) Calories: 125; Total fat: 14g; Saturated fat: 2g; Carbohydrates: <1g; Fiber: 0g; Protein: <1g

KETCHUP

MAKE AHEAD | ONE-POT | PORTABLE | VEGAN Look at the ingredients on a ketchup bottle and you'll see all sorts of things your body just doesn't need, including high fructose corn syrup—a FODMAP enemy. This ketchup is far tastier and you can include your own spice blends to customize it to your personal taste. *Makes 1 cup*

PREP 5 minutes
COOK 10 minutes

2 (6-ounce) cans tomato paste

½ cup apple cider vinegar

¾ teaspoon sea salt

½ teaspoon ground cumin

½ teaspoon ground cinnamon

⅛ teaspoon ground allspice

Pinch ground nutmeg

1. In a medium pot over medium-high heat, combine the tomato paste, cider vinegar, sea salt, cumin, cinnamon, allspice, and nutmeg.

2. Cook for 10 minutes, stirring frequently. Refrigerate in an airtight container for up to 1 week.

for **PLAN A** Tomatoes are not GERD-friendly, so avoid this recipe.

PER SERVING (1 tablespoon) Calories: 20; Total fat: <1g; Saturated fat: 0g; Carbohydrates: 4g; Fiber: 0g; Protein: <1g

BARBECUE SAUCE

MAKE AHEAD | **ONE-POT** | **PORTABLE** | **VEGAN** Building on the earlier Ketchup recipe (page 179), this barbecue sauce is full of goodness without any of the artificial ingredients you find in commercial brands. Fire up the grill! *Makes 1 cup*

PREP 5 minutes
COOK 10 minutes

1 cup Ketchup (page 179)

¼ cup apple cider vinegar

2 tablespoons Garlic Oil (page 184)

4 scallions (green part only), finely chopped

2 tablespoons whiskey (optional)

1 teaspoon chili powder

1 teaspoon smoked paprika

½ teaspoon sea salt

½ teaspoon liquid smoke

⅛ teaspoon freshly ground black pepper

1. In a medium pot over medium-high heat, stir together the ketchup, cider vinegar, garlic oil, scallions, whiskey (if using), chili powder, paprika, sea salt, liquid smoke, and pepper.

2. Cook for 10 minutes, stirring frequently. You can store in the refrigerator in an airtight container for up to 2 weeks, and in the freezer up to 1 year.

for **PLAN A** Tomatoes are not GERD-friendly, so avoid this recipe.

PER SERVING (1 tablespoon) Calories: 20; Total fat: <1g; Saturated fat: 0g; Carbohydrates: 4g; Fiber: 0g; Protein: <1g

BARBECUE RANCH SAUCE

MAKE-AHEAD | **PORTABLE** | **VEGETARIAN** This sauce makes a delicious dip for veggies or snacks, such as the Garlic Parmesan Fries (page 103), the Baked Potato Chips (page 99), or other finger foods. It also makes a tasty topping for burgers. Best of all, it is gut-friendly and packs a powerful flavor punch. *Serves 4*

PREP 5 minutes
COOK 0 minutes

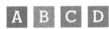

¼ cup Greek yogurt

2 tablespoons Mayonnaise (page 178)

2 tablespoons Barbecue Sauce (page 180)

1 teaspoon Dijon mustard

½ teaspoon lemon zest

½ teaspoon finely chopped fresh dill fronds

½ teaspoon finely chopped fresh chives

¼ teaspoon chili powder

1. In a small bowl, whisk together the yogurt, mayonnaise, barbecue sauce, Dijon mustard, lemon zest, dill, chives, and chili powder until smooth.

2. Refrigerate in an airtight container for up to 5 days.

for **PLAN A** Eliminate the chili powder and chives.

for **PLAN D** Eliminate the chili powder and chives.

PER SERVING (1 tablespoon) Calories: 52; Total fat: 5g; Saturated fat: 1g; Carbohydrates: 3g; Fiber: 1g; Protein: 1g

VEGETABLE BROTH

MAKE AHEAD | ONE-POT | PORTABLE | VEGETARIAN Most commercial broths are made with garlic and onions, so they're generally not FODMAP-friendly. This easy-to-prepare staple cooks on your stove top with little supervision needed, or you can prepare it in a slow cooker for 12 hours on low, which makes it a handy fix-and-forget recipe. *Makes 6 cups*

PREP 5 minutes
COOK 2 hours

 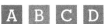

8 cups water

4 carrots, roughly chopped

2 leeks (green part only), roughly chopped

1 celery stalk, chopped

1 fennel bulb, roughly chopped

2 tablespoons Garlic Oil (page 184)

½ teaspoon sea salt

9 peppercorns

1. In a medium pot over medium-high heat, stir together the water, carrots, leeks, celery, fennel, garlic oil, sea salt, and peppercorns. Bring to a boil and reduce the heat to low.

2. Simmer the broth for 2 hours, stirring occasionally. Strain out and discard the solids.

3. Refrigerate in an airtight container for up to 3 days, or freeze for up to 1 year.

for **PLAN A** Eliminate the peppercorns.

PER SERVING (¼ cup) Calories: 38; Total fat: 1g; Saturated fat: 0g; Carbohydrates: <1g; Fiber: 0g; Protein: 4g

POULTRY OR BEEF BROTH

MAKE AHEAD | **ONE-POT** | **PORTABLE** This nutritious broth uses chicken, turkey, or beef bones for flavor. You can simmer it for hours on your stove top, or put it in your slow cooker and walk away. If you use the slow cooker, cook it for 12 to 24 hours on low to develop a rich flavor. *Makes 6 cups*

PREP 5 minutes
COOK 2 hours

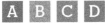

8 cups water

2 pounds chicken, turkey, or beef bones

4 carrots, roughly chopped

2 leeks (green part only), roughly chopped

1 celery stalk, chopped

2 tablespoons Garlic Oil (page 184)

½ teaspoon sea salt

9 peppercorns

1. In a medium pot over medium-high heat, stir together the water, bones, carrots, leeks, celery, garlic oil, sea salt, and peppercorns. Bring to a boil and then reduce the heat to low.

2. Simmer the broth for 2 hours, stirring occasionally. Strain out the solids an discard.

3. Refrigerate in an airtight container for up to 3 days, or freeze for up to 1 year.

for **PLAN A** Eliminate the peppercorns.

PER SERVING (¼ cup) Calories: 38; Total fat: 1g; Saturated fat: 0g; Carbohydrates: <1g; Fiber: 0g; Protein: 4g

GARLIC OIL

MAKE AHEAD | **ONE-POT** | **PORTABLE** | **VEGAN** Love the taste of garlic, but not how it makes you feel? Garlic oil is a great way to infuse garlic flavor into your cooking—without that FODMAP-unfriendly garlic itself. Try it drizzled on a salad, use it for cooking, or add flavor to soup, stews, or anything you love garlic in. You can refrigerate it in an airtight container or freeze it in 1-tablespoon portions in an ice cube tray. *Makes 2 cups*

PREP 5 minutes
COOK 20 minutes, plus
1 hour to steep

2 cups extra-virgin olive oil

8 garlic cloves, peeled and smashed

1. In a medium pot over low heat, combine the olive oil and garlic. Heat for 20 minutes. Remove from the heat and let steep for 1 hour.

2. Strain out the garlic cloves and refrigerate the oil for up to 3 days, or freeze it as described in the headnote for up to 1 year for future use.

for **PLAN A** Garlic may aggravate GERD, so use this recipe with caution.

for **PLAN D** If garlic upsets your stomach, use extra-virgin olive oil in recipes and not this garlic oil.

PER SERVING (1 tablespoon) Calories: 120; Total fat: 14g; Saturated fat: 2g; Carbohydrates: 0g; Fiber: 0g; Protein: 0g

BASIL VINAIGRETTE

MAKE AHEAD | **ONE-POT** | **PORTABLE** | **VEGAN** Vinaigrettes are simple to make, with a basic formula of three parts oil to one part vinegar. With this simple base, you can then infuse any flavors you like. Use about 1 teaspoon of Dijon mustard to help emulsify the vinaigrette. This version features the fresh summery flavor of basil. *Makes 1 cup*

PREP 5 minutes
COOK 0 minutes

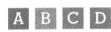

½ cup extra-virgin olive oil

¼ cup Garlic Oil (page 184)

¼ cup apple cider vinegar

¼ cup chopped fresh basil

Zest of 1 lemon

1 teaspoon Dijon mustard

½ teaspoon sea salt

⅛ teaspoon freshly ground black pepper

Pinch red pepper flakes

1. In a medium bowl, whisk together the olive oil, garlic oil, cider vinegar, basil, lemon zest, Dijon mustard, sea salt, black pepper, and red pepper flakes until well combined and emulsified.

2. Refrigerate in an airtight container for up to 1 week.

for **PLAN A** Omit the olive oil and garlic oil. The vinegar in this dressing is not great for GERD, but you can make a creamy version using ¼ cup Mayonnaise (page 178), ¼ cup plain coconut yogurt, 1 tablespoon Dijon mustard, ½ teaspoon sea salt, ¼ cup chopped fresh basil, and the zest of 1 lemon. Whisk to combine.

for **PLAN D** If garlic upsets your stomach, replace the garlic oil with extra-virgin olive oil. Omit the red pepper flakes.

PER SERVING (1 tablespoon) Calories: 91; Total fat: 11g; Saturated fat: 2g; Carbohydrates: 0g; Fiber: 0g; Protein: 0g

ASIAN GINGER VINAIGRETTE

MAKE AHEAD | **ONE-POT** | **PORTABLE** | **VEGAN** This dressing uses Asian spices, so it's great on slaw—among other things. Use a rasp-style grater to grate the ginger very finely. If you can't find Chinese hot mustard powder, don't use jarred mustard because it contains wheat; instead, use 1 teaspoon Dijon mustard. *Makes 1 cup*

PREP 5 minutes
COOK 0 minutes

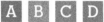

½ cup extra-virgin olive oil

¼ cup Garlic Oil (page 184)

¼ cup apple cider vinegar

¼ cup chopped fresh cilantro

Zest of 1 lime

1 tablespoon grated peeled fresh ginger

1 teaspoon Chinese hot mustard powder

½ teaspoon sea salt

⅛ teaspoon freshly ground black pepper

Pinch red pepper flakes

1. In a medium bowl, whisk the olive oil, garlic oil, cider vinegar, cilantro, lime zest, ginger, mustard powder, sea salt, black pepper, and red pepper flakes until well combined and emulsified.

2. Refrigerate in an airtight container for up to 1 week.

for **PLAN A** Omit the olive oil and garlic oil. The vinegar in this dressing is not great for GERD, but you can make a creamy version using ¼ cup Mayonnaise (page 178), ¼ cup plain coconut yogurt, 1 teaspoon Chinese hot mustard powder, ½ teaspoon sea salt, the zest of 1 lime, ¼ cup chopped fresh cilantro, and 1 tablespoon grated peeled fresh ginger. Whisk to combine.

for **PLAN D** If garlic upsets your stomach, replace the garlic oil with extra-virgin olive oil. Omit the red pepper flakes and Chinese hot mustard powder. Instead substitute 1 teaspoon Dijon mustard.

PER SERVING (1 tablespoon) Calories: 83; Total fat: 10g; Saturated fat: 1g; Carbohydrates: 0g; Fiber: 0g; Protein: 0g

SUNFLOWER BUTTER

MAKE AHEAD | **ONE-POT** | **PORTABLE** | **VEGAN** If you're allergic to peanuts and peanut butter, sunflower butter makes a delicious substitute. You can spread it on gluten-free toast or use it as a dip for fruits and vegetables. You'll need a food processor or blender to make this. *Makes 2 cups*

PREP 5 minutes
COOK 0 minutes

4 cups shelled roasted unsalted sunflower seeds

3 tablespoons coconut oil, melted

¼ cup sugar

Pinch sea salt

1. In a food processor or blender, process the sunflower seeds, coconut oil, sugar, and sea salt on high for 5 to 7 minutes until well blended and creamy in texture.

2. Store in an airtight container at room temperature for 2 to 3 months.

SUBSTITUTION TIP Make this with other nuts and seeds, using the same ratios of nuts to oil to sugar to sea salt.

PER SERVING (1 tablespoon) Calories: 50; Total fat: 4g; Saturated fat: 1g

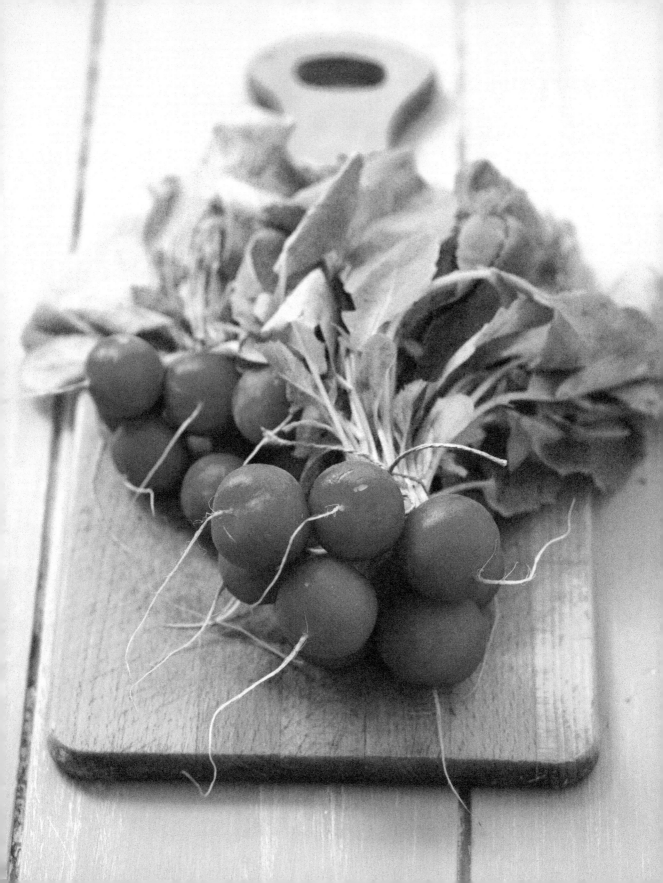

ACKNOWLEDGMENTS

from LAURA

I would like to acknowledge all the wonderful people who helped put this book together: Clara Song Lee, Karen Frazier, and Mary Cassells. It took a lot of coordination and patience to create this book and I am grateful to have been part of this collaboration.

Additionally, I would like to acknowledge all the dietitians out there who have worked so hard to educate the public on the topic of low-FODMAP diets, specifically Sue Shepherd, Kate Scarlata, and Patsy Catsos. They are always ready to share their information and they make our profession a respected field.

from KAREN

I'd like to thank my editor, Clara Song Lee, as well as co-author Laura Manning for the great information provided here.

I'd also like to thank my husband, Jim, and my kids, Kevin and Tanner, for eating whatever I put in front of them—no matter what diet it's a part of—and for their honest feedback.

APPENDIX A
CONVERSION TABLES

VOLUME EQUIVALENTS (LIQUID)

US STANDARD	US STANDARD (OUNCES)	METRIC (APPROXIMATE)
2 tablespoons	1 fl. oz.	30 mL
¼ cup	2 fl. oz.	60 mL
½ cup	4 fl. oz.	120 mL
1 cup	8 fl. oz.	240 mL
1½ cups	12 fl. oz.	355 mL
2 cups or 1 pint	16 fl. oz.	475 mL
4 cups or 1 quart	32 fl. oz.	1 L
1 gallon	128 fl. oz.	4 L

OVEN TEMPERATURES

FAHRENHEIT	CELSIUS (APPROXIMATE)
250°F	120°C
300°F	150°C
325°F	165°C
350°F	180°C
375°F	190°C
400°F	200°C
425°F	220°C
450°F	230°C

VOLUME EQUIVALENTS (DRY)

US STANDARD	METRIC (APPROXIMATE)
⅛ teaspoon	0.5 mL
¼ teaspoon	1 mL
½ teaspoon	2 mL
¾ teaspoon	4 mL
1 teaspoon	5 mL
1 tablespoon	15 mL
¼ cup	59 mL
⅓ cup	79 mL
½ cup	118 mL
⅔ cup	156 mL
¾ cup	177 mL
1 cup	235 mL
2 cups or 1 pint	475 mL
3 cups	700 mL
4 cups or 1 quart	1 L

WEIGHT EQUIVALENTS

US STANDARD	METRIC (APPROXIMATE)
½ ounce	15 g
1 ounce	30 g
2 ounces	60 g
4 ounces	115 g
8 ounces	225 g
12 ounces	340 g
16 ounces or 1 pound	455 g

THE DIRTY DOZEN AND THE CLEAN FIFTEEN

A nonprofit environmental watchdog organization called Environmental Working Group (EWG) looks at data supplied by the US Department of Agriculture (USDA) and the Food and Drug Administration (FDA) about pesticide residues. Each year it compiles a list of the best and worst pesticide loads found in commercial crops. You can use these lists to decide which fruits and vegetables to buy organic to minimize your exposure to pesticides, and which produce is considered safe enough to buy conventionally. This does not mean they are pesticide-free, though, so wash these fruits and vegetables thoroughly.

These lists change every year, so make sure you look up the most recent one before you fill your shopping cart. You'll find the most recent lists, as well as a guide to pesticides in produce, at EWG.org/FoodNews.

DIRTY DOZEN

Apples	Strawberries
Celery	Sweet bell peppers
Cherries	Tomatoes
Cherry tomatoes	*In addition to the Dirty*
Cucumbers	*Dozen, the EWG added*
Grapes	*two types of produce*
Nectarines	*contaminated with highly*
Peaches	*toxic organophosphate*
Spinach	*insecticides:*
	Kale/Collard greens
	Hot peppers

CLEAN FIFTEEN

Asparagus	Kiwis
Avocados	Mangos
Cabbage	Onions
Cantaloupe	Papayas
Cauliflower	Pineapples
Eggplant	Sweet corn
Grapefruit	Sweet peas (frozen)
Honeydew Melon	

REFERENCES

American College of Gastroenterology. "Possible Overlap of IBS Symptoms and Inflammatory Bowel Disease." *ScienceDaily*. October 22, 2012. Accessed July 27, 2016. www.sciencedaily.com /releases/2012/10/121022081236.htm.

Bolen, Barbara, PhD. "What Is IBS-A?" Very Well. Updated June 15, 2016. Accessed July 27, 2016. www.verywell .com/ibs-a-alternating-type-irritable -bowel-syndrome-1944882.

Dibaise, John K., Rosemary J. Young, and Jon A. Vanderhoof. "Enteric Microbial Flora, Bacterial Overgrowth, and Short-Bowel Syndrome." *Clinical Gastroenterology and Hepatology* 4, no. 1 (January 2006): 11–20.

Gibson, Peter R., and Susan J. Shepherd. "Evidence-Based Dietary Management of Functional Gastrointestinal Symptoms: The FODMAP Approach." *Journal of Gastroenterology and Hepatology* 25, no. 2 (2010): 252–58.

International Foundation for Functional Gastrointestinal Disorders. "Facts about IBS." Accessed July 27, 2016. www .aboutibs.org/facts-about-ibs.html.

International Foundation for Functional Gastrointestinal Disorders. "IBS with Constipation." Accessed July 27, 2016. www.aboutibs.org/ibs-with-constipation .html.

International Foundation for Functional Gastrointestinal Disorders. "IBS with Diarrhea." Accessed July 27, 2016. www.aboutibs.org/ibs-with-diarrhea.html.

International Foundation for Functional Gastrointestinal Disorders. "Introduction to IBS." Accessed July 27, 2016. www .aboutibs.org/what-is-ibs-sidenav/intro -to-ibs.html.

Johnson, Kate. "Food Allergies Tied to Irritable Bowel Syndrome." WebMD. Accessed July 27, 2016. www .webmd.com/ibs/news/20151112 /food-allergies-ibs-diarrhea.

Kennedy, Paul J., John F. Cryan, Timothy G. Dinan, and Gerard Clarke. "Irritable Bowel Syndrome: A Microbiome-Gut -Brain Axis Disorder?" *World Journal of Gastroenterology* 20, no. 39 (October 2014): 14105–14125. doi:10.3748 /wjg.v20.i39.14105.

Monash University. "The Monash University Low-FODMAP Diet." Accessed July 27, 2016. www.med.monash.edu/cecs/gastro/fodmap/low-high.html.

National Institutes of Health/National Institute of Diabetes and Digestive and Kidney Diseases. "Short Bowel Syndrome." Accessed July 27, 2016. www.niddk.nih.gov/health-information/health-topics/digestive-diseases/short-bowel-syndrome/Pages/facts.aspx.

Stanisic, Vladimir, and Eamonn M. Quigley. "The Overlap Between IBS and IBD—What Is It and What Does It Mean?" *Expert Review of Gastroenterology & Hepatology* 8, no. 2 (February 2014): 139–45. doi:10.1586/17474124.2014.876361.

Yarandi, Shadi Sadeghi, Siavosh Nasseri-Moghaddam, Pardis Mostajabi, and Reza Malekzadeh. "Overlapping Gastroesophageal Reflux Disease and Irritable Bowel Syndrome: Increased Dysfunctional Symptoms." *World Journal of Gastroenterology* 16, no. 10 (March 2010): 1232–1238. doi:10.3748/wjg.v16.i9.1232

RESOURCES

ONLINE AND APPS

Crohn's and Colitis Foundation of America:
ccfa.org

FODMAP-Friendly:
http://fodmapfriendly.com/app/

IBS Diets:
www.ibsdiets.org/fodmap-diet
/fodmap-food-list/

IBS Factsheet:
http://womenshealth.gov/publications
/our-publications/fact-sheet/irritable
-bowel-syndrome.html

**International Foundation for Functional
Gastrointestinal Disorders:**
www.aboutibs.org

**Irritable Bowel Syndrome Self Help
and Support Group:**
www.ibsgroup.org

Kate Scarlata FODMAP Resources:
www.katescarlata.com

**Low-FODMAP Diet for Irritable Bowel
Syndrome from Monash University:**
www.med.monash.edu/cecs/gastro
/fodmap/

Monash University Low-FODMAP Blog:
http://fodmapmonash.blogspot.com

**Monash University Low-FODMAP
smartphone app:**
www.med.monash.edu.au/cecs/gastro
/fodmap/iphone-app.html

**SIBO (Small Intestine Bacterial Growth)
Specific Foodguide App:**
www.siboinfo.com/apps.html

BOOKS

Scarlata, Kate. *Low-FODMAP 28-Day Plan:
A Healthy Cookbook with Gut-Friendly
Recipes for IBS Relief.* Berkeley, CA:
Rockridge Press, 2014.

Sonoma Press. *The Quiet Gut Cookbook:
135 Easy Low-FODMAP Recipes to Soothe
Symptoms of IBS, ID, and Celiac Disease.*
Berkeley, CA: Sonoma Press, 2015.

Storr, Martin. *The FODMAP Navigator:
Low-FODMAP Diet Charts with Ratings of
More Than 500 Foods, Food Additives, and
Prebiotics.* Seattle: CreateSpace, 2015.

RECIPE INDEX

INDEX

ABOUT THE AUTHORS

LAURA MANNING is a registered dietitian in the department of gastroenterology at the Mount Sinai Medical Center in New York, where she has worked since 2001 with patients diagnosed with irritable bowel syndrome (IBS), inflammatory bowel disease (IBD), celiac disease, and other disorders of the GI tract. She is passionate about helping people avoid the pitfalls of fast food, prepared foods, and processed ingredients, which can lead to obesity and chronic disease, and she guides her patients on simple ways to improve their health. Laura has found a niche in helping malnourished people to gain weight in the healthiest way possible. She lives in Manhattan with her husband and two children and has contributed to *The Huffington Post*, *Fitness* magazine, *Everyday Health*, *SheKnows*, and *MindBodyGreen*.

KAREN FRAZIER is a nutrition and fitness expert who specializes in recipe development for restrictive diets and has written several cookbooks for people with various health conditions, including *The Acid Reflux Escape Plan*, *The Hashimoto's Cookbook and Action Plan*, and *The Gastroparesis Cookbook*. Diagnosed with celiac disease and an acute dairy allergy, Karen understands the challenges of eating a restrictive diet that is both healthful and satisfying and has spent years adapting her own family favorite recipes to meet her dietary needs while still pleasing her family's palates.

CPSIA information can be obtained
at www.ICGtesting.com
Printed in the USA
BVOW05s0007180317
478697BV00002B/4/P